SUBLIMINAL MANIPULATION

The Ultimate Guide To Influence Anyone's Mind Through Persuasion, NLP, Body Language, Stoicism, Mind Control, And Dark Psychology

Copyright © 2020 William J. Coleman. All rights reserved.

This document is geared towards providing exact and reliable information in regard to the topic and issue covered. The publication is sold with the idea that the publisher is not required to render accounting, officially permitted, or otherwise, qualified services. If advice is necessary, legal or professional, a practiced individual in the profession should be ordered. - From a Declaration of Principles which was accepted and approved equally by a Committee of the American Bar Association and a Committee of Publishers and Associations.

In no way is it legal to reproduce, duplicate, or transmit any part of this document in either electronic means or in printed format. Recording of this publication is strictly prohibited and any storage of this document is not allowed unless with written permission from the publisher. All rights reserved. The information provided herein is stated to be truthful and consistent, in that any liability, in terms of inattention or otherwise, by any usage or abuse of any policies, processes, or directions contained within is the solitary and utter responsibility of the recipient reader.

Under no circumstances will any legal responsibility or blame be held against the publisher for any reparation, damages, or monetary loss due to the information herein, either directly or indirectly. Respective authors own all copyrights not held by the publisher. The information herein is offered for informational purposes solely and is universal as so. The presentation of the information is without contract or any type of guarantee assurance.

Table of Contents

INTRODUCTION 1

UNDERSTANDING MANIPULATION 5
    WHAT MANIPULATION IS? 5
    EXAMPLES OF MANIPULATION 14
    HOW TO OUTSMART A MANIPULATOR 19

MANIPULATION TECHNIQUES 24
    NLP FOR MANIPULATION 24
    MIND CONTROL TECHNIQUES 34
    EMOTIONAL MANIPULATION 51
    SUBLIMINAL MANIPULATION 53
    THE ART OF PERSUASION 58
    SELF-MANIPULATION 70

HOW TO GET ANYBODY TO DO WHAT YOU WANT 79
    HOW TO WIN TRUST OF A PERSON 79
    FEAR-THEN-RELIEF PROCEDURE 83
    MAKING YOU FEEL GUILTY: SOCIAL EXCHANGE 86

CONCLUSION 91

Introduction

This is What is the first thing that comes to mind when you hear of the term *manipulation*? For many people, manipulation is a faraway phenomenon that happens to other people, and not to themselves. It is highly unlikely that you will be going about your day thinking about manipulation or worrying that others are manipulating you. Yet the truth of the matter is, manipulation is everywhere around us. It is in sales adverts that try to entice you to buy something that you do not need by convincing you that you do need it. It is in the puppy eyes of a lover or child trying to get something out of you. Manipulation is also at play when a passenger is trying to charm a flight attendant into getting a first-class upgrade. In short, manipulation is everywhere in your daily life. The only reason it goes unnoticed is because high chances are that you are not looking out for it. In many cases, it is often so subtle that even if you were looking for it, you would not notice it.

Manipulation, essentially, is a silent, subtle game happening behind the scenes, and you can bet that you are not the main character. The key to becoming the main actor (or at least avoiding the supporting roles a.k.a being the victim) is to understand what manipulation entails. Once you understand this, you will be in a position to recognize it, avoid it and even beat it. At the same time, understanding manipulation will help you to get better at it, if that is your goal. There is nothing wrong with being good at manipulation. In fact, knowing how to manipulate your way through life situations is a surefire way of being successful at a lot of things. The only thing you should be careful of is how you use your newly gained skills. The reason why manipulation often gets such a bad rap is because, in many instances, manipulators use their skills to the detriment of others.

People are often a product of their environment, whether they want to be or not. The way people are raised directly affects the way they act in later life. Someone who is raised by alcoholics has a greater chance of becoming alcoholics in adult life, or they may choose never to drink at all. People who are raised in a house where everything is forbidden may cut loose and go a bit crazy when they are finally out on their own. People who are raised in total disorganization may grow up to be totally obsessive about household cleanliness.

Nurture affects people in other, less severe ways, too. Many people believe that Mom's meatloaf is the absolute best and no other recipe exists. People come from different religious and economic backgrounds. People have different beliefs about what is good and bad, what is acceptable and unacceptable. The problem comes when two people are trying to have a relationship, but neither wants to change their way of thinking. When that happens there is no relationship. There are just two people living together under the same roof.

In our social interactions, we're much more than our inherent mannerisms and idiosyncrasies. We're a world of experiences, cultural presumptions and social constructs. To better understand why people behave the way they do, a good place to start is by examining your own reactions and responsive behaviors in confrontation of the way in which others behave. How do you react to certain situations?

A man is running down the street naked. Do you laugh, or do you scream? Maybe you call the police. Maybe you rip off your clothes and run along with him! Any of these reactions makes perfect sense to the person pursuing them, but which of them is going to seem more normative? That will vary greatly from culture to culture and from person to person. And while our responses to any number of incidents, events, situations and stimuli may be somewhat culturally and socially-mandated, they're also highly individual and also, well within our ability to choose. We're not puppets in a play, controlled by an invisible puppet master who pulls our strings and makes us dance. We choose our responses. We choose our reactions and actions.

While you're going to feel the heat in the kitchen, how you respond to it is a matter of choice. You either mop your brow and carry on, or run for the door, pulling at your clothes; gasping for air. Then again, it is pretty difficult to be sad at the circus! Most people love a good show. Some people, though, fear clowns. Others feel badly for the animals, so while the exception proves the rule, the truth is that our responses are all highly individual.

Your responses are not pre-determined, even though it's pretty easy to predict responses in certain situations (with varying success, as shown above). But if that's so, then you can learn how to tailor your own behavior to present a more unruffled and confident image to others. Ultimately, you are in command of your own responses. By the same token, you are in command of your ability to engage people at a much deeper and more effective level, when you're able to accurately interpret what's going on underneath their words. Remembering that Triplett pointed to the fact that people behave differently in public situations than they do in private ones, we can think of the people around us emotional onions. Just like us, they're full of layers. What the surface tells us can be deceptive, until we begin peeling it back to reveal the next layer and the next, after that.

People have many good reasons for this tendency to conceal the true selves in public. Some of that has to do with trust. Sometimes, they prefer to hide their true natures for fear of not being liked. Other times, they feel it's to their advantage not to show their hand until it's time to play it. For every person on earth, there's a unique set of motivations for the modelling of two faces. This is not necessarily consciously pursued to deceive others. It's more a matter of self-preservation and that's part of the natural, human survival instinct.

Understanding Manipulation

What Manipulation Is?

Manipulation is a form of social influence which uses indirect, underhanded, and deceptive tactics to change people's perceptions and their resultant behavior. Usually, the end goal is to advance the interests of the person who initiates the manipulation. In many cases, manipulation happens at the expense of the person that is being manipulated; they may be emotionally, mentally, or physically harmed, or they may end up taking actions that are against their own best interests.

It's important to note that social influence is not inherently bad; one person can use manipulation techniques for the good of the person he or she is manipulating. For example, your family members or friends can use social influence and manipulation to get you to do something for your own good. The people who mean you well might manipulate you as a way of helping you deal with certain challenges or to help you make the right decisions.

However, in this book, we won't focus on the garden-variety harmless forms of social influence. We are more interested in the kind of manipulation that is done with malicious intentions. This is the kind of manipulation that disregards a person's right to accept or reject influence. It is coercive in nature; when the person being targeted tries to push against it, this kind of manipulation gets more sophisticated, and the end goal is to negate the person's will to assert for themselves.

How Manipulation Works

There are several psychological theories that explain how successful manipulation works. The first and perhaps the most universally accepted theory is one that was put forth by renowned psychologist and author, George Simon. He analyzed the concept of manipulation from the point of view of the manipulator, and he can up with a pattern of behavior that sums up every manipulation scenario. According to Simon, there are three main things that are involved in psychological manipulation.

First, the manipulator approaches the target by concealing his or her aggressive intentions. Here, the manipulator seeks to endear himself to his target without revealing the fact that his ultimate plan is to manipulate him or her. The manipulator accomplishes this by modifying his behavior and presenting himself as a good-natured and friendly individual, one who relates well with the target.

Secondly, the manipulator will take time to know the victim. The purpose of this is to get to understand the psychological vulnerabilities that the victim may have so as to figure out which manipulation tactic will be the most effective when he ultimately decides to deploy them.

Depending on the scenario, and the complexity of the manipulation technique, this stage may take anywhere between a few minutes to several years. For example, when a stranger targets you, he may take only a couple of minutes to "size you up" but when your partner or colleague seeks to manipulate you, he or she may spend months or even years trying to understand how your mind works.

The success of this second step depends on how well the first step is executed. If the manipulator successfully hides his intentions from you, he is in a better position to learn your weaknesses because you will instill some level of trust in him, and he will use that trust to get you to let down your guard and to reveal your vulnerabilities to him.

Thirdly, having collected enough information to act upon, the manipulator will deploy a manipulation technique of his choosing. For this to work, the manipulator needs to be able to marshal a sufficient level of ruthlessness; this means that the manipulation technique chosen will depend on what the manipulator can stomach. A manipulator with a conscience may try to use methods that are less harmful to manipulate you. One that completely lacks a conscious may use extreme methods to take advantage of you. Either way, manipulative people are willing to let harm befall their victims, and to them, the resultant outcome (which is usually in their favor) justifies the harm they cause.

Simon's theory of manipulation teaches us the general approach that manipulators use to get what they want from their victims, but it also points out something extremely important: Manipulation works, not just because of the actions of the manipulator, but also because of the reactions of the victims.

In the first step, the manipulator misrepresents himself to the victim: If the victim is able to see through the veil that the manipulator is wearing, the manipulation won't be successful. In the second step, the manipulator collects information about victims to learn about his or her vulnerabilities. The victim can be may be able to stop the manipulation at this stage by treating the manipulator's prying nature with a bit of suspicion. In the third stage, the manipulator uses coercive or underhanded techniques to get what he wants from the victim. Even in this stage, the victim may have certain choices on how to react to the manipulator's machinations.

The point here is that when it comes to manipulation, it takes two to tango. By understanding both the victim's and the manipulator's psychology, it's possible to figure out how you can avoid falling victim to other people's manipulation, and it can also help you become more conscientious so that you don't unknowingly use manipulation techniques on other people around you.

Let's look at the vulnerabilities that manipulators like to exploit in their victims.

The first and most prevalent vulnerability is the need to please others. We all have this need to some extent; we seek to please the people in our lives as well as total strangers. This is technically a positive quality that helps us coexist in our societies, but to manipulators, it's a weapon that can be used against you.

Many of us are willing to endure certain levels of discomfort just to make other people feel happy; we feel a certain sense of obligation towards one another, and that's just human nature. The closer we are to certain people, the greater the need to please them. For example, the need to please your friend is higher than your need to please a stranger.

Manipulators understand this, and they use it against their victims all the time. If a manipulator wants to get something big out of you, he will first take the time to get closer to you, not just to get to know your vulnerability, but also to increase the sense of obligation you feel towards him.

The second vulnerability is the need for approval and acceptance. Again, as social beings, we all have an innate desire to feel accepted. We want people to love us, to think of us as members of their groups, and to choose us over other people. This feeling can be addictive, and it can give other people (especially manipulative ones) a lot of power over us. The vast majority of manipulation victims are people who have close personal relationships with the manipulators; in other words, they have an emotional need to gain the acceptance or approval of the manipulator. The remaining manipulation victims can be manipulated because they want to be a part of something (a group, a social class, etc.).

The third vulnerability that manipulators like to exploit is what psychologists refer to as "emetophobia" (which is the fear of negative emotions). To some extent, we are all afraid of negative emotions; we will do lots of things to avoid feeling angry, afraid, stressed, frustrated, and worried, etc. We want to lead happy and fulfilled lives, and anything that makes us feel "bad" is a threat to that sense of fulfillment. So, in many cases, we will do what manipulators want if it serves to alleviate that "bad" feeling. Manipulators know this, and they use negative emotions against us all the time.

The fourth vulnerability is the lack of assertiveness. Assertiveness is a very rare quality; even people who you may generally consider to be assertive are likely to cave in if manipulators push hard enough. Even when you are willing to stand your ground and to say "No," manipulators can be very persistent, and in the end, they can wear you out.

The fifth vulnerability is the lack of a strong sense of identity. Having a strong sense of identity means having clear personal boundaries, and understanding one's own values. Unfortunately, these qualities aren't so strong in most of us, and that leaves us open to manipulation. Manipulators succeed by pushing our boundaries little by little, making them blurry, and then taking control of our identities.

Finally, having an external locus of control, and having a low level of self-reliance are also key vulnerabilities that manipulators love to exploit. When you have an external locus of control, it means that your identity and your sense of self are external to you. It means you view yourself through other people's eyes. It means that you are extrinsically motivated. When you have low self-reliance, it means you depend on other people for sustenance and for emotional stability. It means that if support systems in your life are taken away, you can easily find yourself leaning on a manipulator, which leaves you at his mercy.

Manipulation is a Part of Human History

Looking at history, we will see that some of our most loved historical figures practiced manipulation. During the founding of the United States, our founding fathers had to use socio-political manipulation to help set a revolution in motion. By first using various economic manipulation tactics on the other colonies and colonists that joining their cause would benefit them more than say the British. Secondly, among each other many political games had to be played, all using subterfuge and manipulation to help get the right people in place to lead the country.

Manipulation had to be used in its persuasive form here so that the right person could get the right backing. This was not evil nor bad; it showed how the covert tactic of playing into a willing pawns card could allow for everyone involved to win. Imagine, too, that they had to manipulate the British for quite a while before things truly were sent into emotion. They had to manipulate them into trusting and believing them. These same kinds of manipulative games have been used for good by many great figures in history to simply manipulate their opposition into doing what is right.

Think of the rallies and marches during the civil rights movement. It did so much good by manipulating and playing on people's emotions and wants for a just society. This is not malicious manipulation, but more so an evil required to enact great change in this world.

Knowing that manipulation is not always an evil wantonly committed for evil makes it much easier to understand the kind of tactics people will use. In a big part complimenting and persuading someone through charisma is, in a sense, manipulation. You are telling them what they want to hear whether it compliments or being a shoulder to cry on for someone.

Almost every friendship that is healthy has this give and take. For a large part, these are simple altruistic forms of manipulation that allow and help both sides win and accomplish a goal of theirs. Charisma and persuasion two topics I mentioned earlier. Persuasion and charisma are the simplest forms of human manipulation.

Manipulators work by making someone come across as if they are the type of person who loves and cares about you and would drop anything if need be to help you with something. This glib or charm is a manipulative tactic that one could use for themselves to try and gain friends. Once again, there is nothing wrong with this; its more in line with gaming the system. You are putting on a front that people want, and as a result of this, they then become drawn to you easier and wish to spend time with you or do stuff to you.

This is a simple day to day manipulation that we all do – whether we realize it or not. This type of manipulation on a social scale is not for harm, but for companionship. Have you ever heard the expression "a little white lie"? The issue is that the word makes manipulation sound bad and evil. But the truth is that by doing simple things that social charmer does, like mirroring body language, buying someone food, or always asking about their interests and ignoring yours is basic human interaction. You can get people to trust you and even help you get ahead in life, especially if this kind of interaction is taking place in the social world.

Manipulation and Success

You could argue that to a certain degree without some powerful people in society who used manipulation to get their way to the top, the world would fall apart. Maybe we would not be so successful. This kind of manipulation is far more different than the much more sinister mind manipulation. It is simple to understand the term mental manipulation. Simply put, mental manipulation occurs with the nefarious act of playing mind games, such as making you feel guilty for not buying or doing something, getting you to question your own judgment.

This covert manipulative behavior can become so common that we oftentimes don't recognize it until it is too late by which point, we have befallen the consequences of said manipulation. Avoiding these consequences is a great thing to be capable of doing. But it can be hard to avoid if you are not sure what you are avoiding. Well, that is why it is good to know what mental manipulation is due to its subtlety. It is this type of manipulation – mental manipulation – which is perhaps the most common form of manipulation you will encounter in your day to day life.

Mental manipulation shows its face a lot in relationships with friends or other people you care about. As a result, the people who do this are very good at it and hide it well. Besides being such a common form of manipulation people will use, it is important to realize that there are many varieties of mental manipulation to which you could easily find yourself as a victim.

Consider times when you are speaking with a group of friends, and one person tries to make you feel guilty due to you making a choice to not buy them an extremely expensive gift for their birthday. They then might try mental manipulation to get you to fall for the trap of "oh well, I have done all these things for you; do you not think it is fair if you get me xyz."

Behavior like this is where manipulation becomes evil and unacceptable. This is not trying to sway someone over to your side of thinking for a good reason or trying to survive in a time of crisis. This narcissistic person is using manipulation to hurt people, and that is never acceptable.

Understanding the subtle moral differences in manipulation makes it easier for you to appreciate how to learn about different manipulative tactics as a whole and how you yourself can go about defending from and using them as well as giving you the useful ability of knowing how to avoid people who could potentially try and manipulate you in person, this includes the media and everything else we see. Since they all use manipulation tactics, understanding this is half the battle.

Examples of Manipulation

Body language is a potent tool needed for mastering how to manipulate people. If you can honestly understand how body language works and be able to analyze it, then you will be in control of the other person, though in a tactical manner.

The way body language works as a compass is by telling you very important things about how the person is feeling and what they are thinking in the present. This information will help you understand how they feel about their environment and what is going on around them, as well as how they feel about you and their interactions with you, or anyone else with whom they may be sharing interactions. Knowing this information means that you have an incredible upper hand when it comes to interacting with the person. With it, you now know when you should approach them and how, which manipulation and persuasion strategies you should use, what wording would likely work best on them, and even the exact timing of when you should be able to completely tip them in your favor.

As you can clearly tell, body language is an essential compass in helping you effectively manipulate people. This is the very first step before you move toward anything else. For that reason, it is vital that you understand the "reading formula," or how you will assess the three types of body language that you will be reading on the person in front of you. This formula is basic, and can even be crafted into an easy-to-remember sentence, just like the one you use to remember the three steps of manipulation.

As you now know, basic body language is the part of the body language you are reading to get a general understanding of what a person is thinking and feeling at the moment. This is the first thing you want to read before you approach a person or begin manipulating them, as this will give you an understanding of where they stand and what path you need to take to get to where you want to go. After you have gained this general understanding, you typically do not want to find yourself focused excessively on basic body language.

When you are reading complex body language signals, you want to look at two primary areas: their hands and their feet. The location and actions being taken with these two parts of the body will tell you more than almost anywhere else on the entire body.

By reading the signs being given to you by the hands and feet, you can get an idea of what the person is thinking and how they are feeling. In general, you want to watch the movements taking place in the hands and feet during your conversation with the person you are talking to and wanting to manipulate. Use them to determine whether you are successfully driving the person into the emotion that you need them to be in for manipulation to happen, or if you need to adjust your tactics to get them there. Pay attention to them during the course of the entire conversation, especially when you use a specific manipulation tactic. These complex signals will act as a form of compass to guide you through the conversation step-by-step, on their terms that are secretly orchestrated by you.

Let us analyze some of the possible ways a person can manipulate others using his body language.

Manipulation by Mirroring the Other Person

When you consciously and deliberately change your body language to fit into another person's class and even behave like the person by learning the tone of voice, posture, facial expressions, including micro-expressions. This merely is mimicry or imitation aimed at impressing someone else.

Although, this process could be risky because the other person may get to know you are just trying to make a false impression and it could cost you the relationship or other valuable details. It is better to maintain your natural body language than mirroring another person's traits, which has the potentials of backfiring at the end, leaving you in pieces.

Exciting and Captivating their Emotions

This step is a beneficial method of manipulating people easily by exciting and captivating their minds through their emotions. Finding out the issue troubling their heart and using it as bait in luring them into doing what will be an advantage to you.

Make People to Like You

You may want to ask me, what shall I do to make people like me? No matter the intrigues and tactics, you want to use in manipulating people, it may not work if they don't like you naturally. Therefore, endeavor to make yourself a likable person. The character is one of the criteria that will cause people to quickly and gullibly accept whatever you say to them. Howbeit, remember that your ultimate goal is to make everything work to your advantage, nothing less than that.

Present Yourself as a Trustworthy Person

Trust is the crucial thing in every relationship. If your friend does not trust you, he will not commit salient details to you. One of the criteria to win the trust of your friend is to share a very private issue with him or her, and that will make him open his or her heart for you too. With this gesture, you may win the confidence of your partner, as he is poised to confide in you.

Use Your Emotions to manipulate them

The very first step to analyzing anyone is to analyze their body language. Body language is something that virtually every master manipulator has learned how to read, and it is essential that you learn how, too. Body language is a level of language that we use to communicate beyond the spoken word. You have likely heard about, and maybe even learned about body language in the past. Still, it is vital that you understand how to read body language from a manipulator's point of view if you want to effectively analyze a person.

Set a Baseline

When you have a baseline about people, reading body language and other nonverbal clues becomes more accurate. Tune in to people completely to figure out their baseline or essential behavior. This will help you relate nonverbal clues more effectively. How does someone react to different circumstances and situations? What is their inherent personality? How are their communication skills? How is their speech and choice of words? What about the voice? Are they essentially confident or anxious?

Look for a Group of Clues

Read clues in clusters, which offer a more accurate analysis of what a person is thinking or feeling. Do not make quick and sporadic conclusions based on isolated nonverbal signals.

Spotting Lies and Deception

While reading people for deception, it is crucial to keep their baseline behavior and the physical setting and culture/religion into context too. Reading or analyzing people through body language is not an overnight process, but it keeps getting accurate with practice. Try deciphering what people are thinking or feeling by practicing people reading skills at the airport, in the train to work, at the doctor's clinic, or cafe. You'll learn to tune in to their actions and behavior accurately over a period of time.

General Body Language Signs

If you are speaking and someone is leaning in your direction, he or she is clearly interested in what you are saying or keenly listening to you. Likewise, crossed arms and legs are a huge sign of switching off or being completely closed to what you are trying to communicate. The person does not really subscribe to your views or isn't confident about what you are saying. Sometimes, people offer wide smiles yet cross their arms while listening to you.

Smile

This information can be extremely valuable considering smile is the single largest weapon people use to conceal their real thoughts, emotions, and feelings. It is a widely established conclusion among psychological experts that a smile is tough to fake. There has to be a genuine experience of joy or happiness for creating that specific expression. When you aren't really happy, the expressions will not settle into their place.

How to Outsmart a Manipulator

Psychological manipulation is always going to be a very loaded and heavy-handed issue. It can often be referred to as lying, deceiving, skewing, distorting, gaslighting, intimidating, guilting, and other such things. Manipulators can also take the form of many different people over the course of your life. Sometimes, the person who is manipulating you might be a parent, sibling, boss, classmate, coworker or romantic partner, among others. That's why manipulation is such a complex topic to handle. It can take the form of various tactics, and it can also be employed by various agents. This is why it can be increasingly difficult for someone to be able to identify and deal with a manipulative person.

You were exposed to the many different feelings, sensations, and experiences that you might have should you ever find yourself in a manipulative relationship environment. As long as you keep your eyes peeled and you make an active effort in seeking these red flags out, it shouldn't really be a problem. Now, it's a matter of dealing with these people and managing their advances.

First evaluate whether the person is more of a systematic or unconscious manipulator. The more systematic, profound manipulators are almost certainly beyond reach. They can have grand visions and don't care who they have to get by to pursue their goals, they may simply enjoy controlling others, perhaps they have had childhood traumas and issues that lead them to exploit others for fulfillment. These types of people are more aware of it and aggressively pursue their manipulative traits. Whatever the case may be, if possible, keep your distance on these types of people. Indeed, the easy solution would be to cut this person out of your life, right?

It can be so easy to just burn bridges with someone if you know that they have manipulative tendencies and that they would be so willing to advance their own personal interests at your expense. That kind of selfishness should warrant a cutting of ties. However, it's not always going to be that simple. There are going to be times when the person who is manipulating you is someone you have a deep bond and connection with. There is even a chance they are not consciously aware of their behavior themselves. For instance, if your parent, partner or friend is manipulating you, it's not going to be so easy to just break that relationship off entirely. This is especially true if you love your parents and you know that they love you in return. In this case, it's not just a matter of eliminating a manipulative person from your life. Rather, it becomes an issue of managing this individual.

When dealing with a manipulative person, it's very important that you tread lightly. Keep in mind that there is also a paternal kind of manipulation. They might not have bad intentions, and they might take offense to the fact that you are accusing them of being manipulative. That is why you have to be extra cautious and sensitive when you broach the issue with them.

First, Be Safe

If you know that you are in danger whenever you are with this manipulative individual in your life, always make sure that there is a third-party present. You can never really know what they might do to you if the two of you are alone. So, before you confront them about your manipulation, make sure that you have someone else in the room. You need that mediator; someone who would be able to help bridge the two of you. You can always call on a mutual friend, a shared loved one, or a trusted confidante. In more serious cases, you can even seek professional help from a licensed therapist. The point here is that the confrontation process should never be conducted recklessly. Your safety is always going to be the first priority here. And a lot of the time, that means having someone else in the room to be with you.

Take a Diplomatic Approach to Initiating a Dialogue

You can either choose to work your own influence on them to lessen the negative effects, or you could just confront them. The initial confrontation doesn't have to be so hot and impassioned. In fact, the best approach to confronting this individual would be to be as calm and collected as can be. You want to make sure that you are taking emotions out of the equation here. Keep in mind that a manipulative person is always going to capitalize on the emotionality of a person. If you take that ammo away from them, then it leaves them very little to work with. In addition to that, it's more likely that they won't react in such a hostile manner if you take a more civil approach to initiating this dialogue with them. Using people's own words against them makes it harder to resist whatever it is you are asking them to do, if one claims to be selfless, then they would not partake in certain actions to begin with.

You have to remember that starting the conversation isn't always going to go so smoothly. It's very much likely that they will resist at first. However, you need to stay persistent. You have to emphasize the importance of this conversation. However, if they do decide to engage with you in this conversation, then you need to stay mindful of the following tips.

Don't Fight Back

If they are going to be hostile with you about it, resist the urge to fight back. You have to learn to pick your spots. Responding to them in a hostile manner is only going to result in you playing into their games. You don't want that. You want to make sure that you stay calm all throughout. When they get emotional, don't invalidate these feelings. Their emotions might actually be very authentic regardless of whether they are based on distorted truths or not. A person can still feel angry about something that is a complete lie or fantasy. Keep that in mind.

Instead of invalidating their feelings and telling them that they're being unreasonable, hear them out. With this method, you will get a chance to really understand them more. You will be able to gain insight into their behavioral triggers. The more you understand them, then the better it will be for you to manage this entire situation.

Set Clear Limits and Boundaries

Once you have heard their side of the tale, it's now time for you to air out your personal grievances. Again, you need to make sure that you keep emotions out of it. You don't want them to be invalidating what you're saying just because you're being hysterical. You want to be honest about it, and be straight. You shouldn't be beating around the bush anymore. Make sure that all of the skeletons come out of the closet. Be courteous, but also, don't pull any punches. No matter how uncomfortable it might be to speak honestly about your feelings, you're going to have to do so.

If you're interested in salvaging the relationship, then emphasize this point. Make sure they understand that you don't want to block them out of your life completely. However, you also need to emphasize that you will be setting clear limits and boundaries as you move forward in your relationship together. Make them understand that the integrity of your relationship is dependent on their respect for the boundaries that you set in it.

Know When It's Time to Walk Away

Sometimes, you just need to be able to know when it's time to walk away. No matter how painful it is to cut yourself loose from someone who you love dearly, you still have to do so for the sake of your own well-being. You should not be making any room for toxicity or manipulative behavior that causes burden in your life regardless of who it might be coming from. At the end of the day, the only real person who has your back is yourself. That is why you have to make it a point to protect yourself at all costs. If there is no way for you to find a peaceful means of coexisting with one another that doesn't involve any form of harmful manipulation that is taking value out of your life, then you need to be able to walk away from that.

Granted, walking away from someone who is close to you isn't going to be a quick and easy process. It's going to be a very painful and gradual one. However, you always need to prioritize your own well-being above the relationships that you have with others, especially if they are the toxic and systematic type. Stay safe and guarded. No relationship is worth losing your sense of self over.

Manipulation Techniques

NLP for Manipulation

Here, we will look at NLP techniques that can be used to influence others in social situations and in ordinary interpersonal dynamics. Here, we will discuss techniques that use those concepts to help you get what you want.

Embedding Commands in the Statements That You Make

When you want someone to comply with a request that you are making, you can make statements in such a way that they include specific commands.

For instance, if you want to ask your friend to schedule a lunch date with you, you can phrase your request as a command instead of a question. So, instead of saying, "can we have lunch sometime this week?" you say "let's have lunch this week."

It may seem like the same request either way, but the reactions you'll get from those two statements are completely different. The first one is a question, so there is room for a yes or no answer. Here, your friend is highly likely to turn you down even if scheduling your lunch date is only slightly inconvenient.

When you say "let's have lunch this week," it feels like a commanding statement. This kind of phrasing primes your friend to feel as though the question of whether or not you are going to have lunch is a foregone conclusion, and now the only thing that's left, is for the two of you to figure out the logistics. So, in his mind turning you down is going to feel like an insurmountable task, and he will be more inclined to adjust his schedule to accommodate your lunch date.

There is also a greater sense of urgency in the second request that there is in the first one. Even if your friend is generally inclined to have lunch with you at some point in the future, the first request increases the chances that your friend will try to bargain and schedule your date further away. The second request, on the other hand, creates the impression that the date needs to happen as soon as possible, so in your friend's mind, it will register as a major priority.

There are many other ways that you can conceal commands in the statements that you make. This is especially done in sales and marketing; salespeople are trained to use hidden commands to upsell you when you go to their stores. For example, when you've just bought a shiny new electronic gadget, if you are dealing with a well-trained salesperson she will ask you "what accessories do you want with that?" instead of "do you want any accessories with that?"

In the first statement, there is the implication that you have to get at least one or more accessories, but in the second statement, there is the implication that accessories are generally optional. If you have a few bucks left, you are more likely to consider spending them on an accessory if you heard the first question than you are likely to do it if you heard the second question.

Creating the Illusion of Choice

The illusion of choice is also a common NLP technique, and it can be used to condition someone to select a specific option (or one option from a limited set of choices) while conditioning him to think that he has several choices at his disposal. The illusion of choice can be used in romantic relationships, in parenting, in the workplace, and in lots of other social dynamics.

For example, let's say you walk into a restaurant, and you get seated, then your waiter walks over and asks "which wine would you like, red or white?" you might go ahead, check the wine list, and order something that's within your price range. However, if the waiter comes over and asks, "What would you like to drink?" or "would you like some wine?" you would be more inclined to turn him down.

The difference here is that in the first instance, the waiter has limited your options, and he has primed you to think that you have a choice. You will be choosing whether or not you want a red or white wine, and you may even have to choose between different brands and different price points. Since you are presented with a fixed set of choices, your mind still thinks that you are acting on your own free will, so you don't feel as though you have been manipulated.

On the other hand, when the waiter asks what you would like to drink, or if you would like some wine, your options aren't restricted. So, mentally, you wouldn't feel at all uncomfortable if you just asked for some water, or if you ordered a cocktail instead.

Some savvy marketing experts can add a twist to the illusion of choice technique to make people more inclined to select one option over another. If for instance, there are two things to pick from, and a salesperson wants you to pick the one that profits him the most, he may introduce a third "decoy option" to steer you towards the choice he wants.

For example, restaurant menus often sell combined items at a lower price than they do individual items to make people think that they are getting a bargain when they order more items.

For example, a restaurant may lists its menu items as follows: Burger -- $2.30; Fries -- $1.50; Burger & Fries -- $3.30. Now supposing you walked into the restaurant planning only to have a burger. Once you look over the menu, you realize that you will "save" $0.50 if you selected the combo instead.

Strategic Use of the Words "but" & "and"

These two words may seem simple, but they have a lot of weight when they are strategically used in conversation.

You can use the word "and" at the beginning of all your sentences during the conversation to indicate agreeableness and to prime the other person to be more agreeable by extension. The "and game" is often used in improvisational theatre to help people generate free-flowing ideas, but in interpersonal conversations, you can use an iteration of that game to make the other person feel like they can open up to you.

It's very simple; when someone is done speaking, follow up their last sentence with the word "and," then add your own statement. For example, if your date says, "This steak is really delicious," you can follow that with "and it pairs well with this wine." This creates the impression that your minds are in sync, so the person will be more receptive to your ideas.

The word "but" on the other hand has the power to negate anything that comes before it in a sentence and to make the listener lend more weight on whatever comes after.

Let's take these two sentences as examples: If your friend told you "my brother is a very smart guy, but he can be difficult to deal with." you are more likely to think that her brother might not make great company because you will have a difficult time dealing with him.

However, if your friend says "My brother can be difficult to deal with, but he is a very smart guy" you are more likely to think that her brother might provide interesting company, and getting along with him might be slightly challenging at first.

The phrase that comes afterward seems to hold more significance than the one that comes before; so you can keep that in mind in cases where you have to deliver both positive and negative news, or in scenarios where you have to talk about something's negative and positive qualities.

For example, if you are selling a second-hand car, you are more likely to win over a customer by saying "the rear has a slight bump, but it gets good gas mileage" instead of saying "it gets good gas mileage, but the rear has a slight bump."

Reframing

Reframing is an NLP technique that is most commonly used by salespeople to get their customers to change the way they perceive things. One of the most effective ways to change a person's mind is by altering their perception – reframing is the process that goes into altering people's perceptions.

Reframing involves taking a fact, a belief or conviction, and restating it so that your target sees the situation from an angle that he has never considered before. Reframing is a way of changing the meaning of something, so that it becomes more powerful or less powerful, depending on what it is you want to get out of the situation. Reframing often involves redefining something that your target things of as a problem, and making it seem like a challenge.

For example, when someone tells you, "Your idea is stupid." You can reframe that situation by saying, "Yeah, but it's also stupid not to consider all possibilities." In this case, you have taken the person's fear of seeming stupid, turned it around, and used it against him. So, in his mind, he feels like he will be betraying his own logic if he doesn't consider your idea.

NLP experts who work in sales often use the concept of "disruptive reframing" to make their products, services, and ideas seem more valuable to potential clients. Disruptive reframing refers to a persuasion technique where the audience's focus is shifted or disrupted in a way that makes certain things seem more manageable.

Disruptive reframing is often used in car adverts. For example, instead of saying that a car costs $15,000, the dealer may state that it costs "$3000 per year" or "$250 per month." A more creative dealer may break it down further by claiming that the same car costs $8 per day. He might even try to completely change the frame and take money out of the equation by claiming that you can get the car "for the price of two cups of coffee per day."

In this example, the salesperson isn't lying; he is just reframing the facts in a disruptive way. He knows that a $15,000 price tag may seem intimidating for a person with an average income and many expenses, so he takes away his customers' concerns by equating that amount of money to something small that people spend money on without thinking twice.

Having the Last Word in a Discussion

The last words are extremely powerful. There is a reason why people are obsessed with "famous last words" of historical figures. Just like those famous last words sum up the lives of great men and women in history, the last word in a conversation sums up the entire conversation. Even if you had differing opinions during a conversation, and even if you "agreed to disagree" with the other person, having the last word makes your point stronger in his or her mind.

Some people tend to let others have the last word in arguments because they just want the argument to end, but that is unwise. Manipulators who understand NLP can use last words to steer you in the direction in which they want you to go.

Even in casual talks, manipulative people will insist on saying the last thing because, from an anthropological and psychological standpoint, it somehow implies that they are higher than the other person in the dominance hierarchy, and therefore their word carries more weight. Think about formal settings (such as boardroom meetings, political rallies, etc.), the highest-ranking person is almost always the last one to speak, and he or she is the one who dismisses the meeting, by literary giving others permission to leave the room and go out and do something else.

You can use NLP to exert dominance over somebody in the long run by having the last word every time you talk to them. If you hold collegial meetings with your coworkers (those who are at your peer level), you can create the impression that you are the "alpha" of the group by always being the one that has the last word.

The Use of Questions

NLP experts love this technique because it enables them to hijack someone's thought patterns without them realizing it. Questions are so effective at steering people's thoughts; they are often used in mass media, in political rhetoric, and in many other areas. Questions have a way of forcing the target to look at things from the point of view of the manipulator.

Questions allow you to make a statement without making it. You may have encountered news headlines like "Are eggs bad for you?" or "Is fossil fuel the only viable energy source?" In such instances, the writers of these articles want to convey a controversial point of view that they have (e.g. "eggs are bad for you" or "the benefits of fossil fuels outweigh the environmental concerns") but because they know that these ideas may face pushback, they choose to present them as questions so that they seem ambiguous.

You can use this technique in interpersonal relationships. For example, if you are trying to talk someone out of a certain idea or point of view, you can do it by saying "You seem to raise some good points, but ask yourself this question." When you drop in the question, your target will have no choice but to ponder on the idea that underlies that question. You have effectively taken control of his thought process, and you have pushed it in a direction that is favorable for you.

Using the Word "Don't"

NLP experts can use the word "don't" as a decoy to steer people's thoughts towards a certain direction in order to influence their emotions and actions.

The human mind has a difficult time comprehending negatives. In many cases, it processes negative statements the exact same way it processes positive statements.

If someone tells you "think about elephants," images of elephants are going to pop into your mind.

If someone else tells you "don't think about lions," images of lions are going to pop into your mind.

While your conscious mind can logically tell the difference between the positive and the negative statement, your subconscious mind cannot (remember that the subconscious uses a different linguistic system). So if you tell someone not to focus on something, he will inevitably focus on it.

You can use the word "don't" as an NLP technique in almost all areas in life. If you want to nudge your spouse into thinking about your future plans subliminally, you can mention in passing how lucky you are that you don't have to think about those plans for a while.

For example, if you want your spouse to start thinking about buying a home, you can just pretend to be reading the business section of a newspaper and say something like "It looks like the housing market is still recovering. I'm glad we don't have to think about buying a home for now."

When you say that, your spouse won't be able to help it; he will start thinking about buying the house because that's what his subconscious mind will tell him to do.

Using the Word "Means"

Our brains are wired to find meaning in the information that we take in and find links and associations between different ideas and concepts. This is crucial for our survival; the brain creates "maps of meaning" for the sensory information that we gather so that when we encounter that information, later on, we know exactly what we are dealing with. this explains why children as so inquisitive; for the brain to function properly, everything we encounter needs to hold some meaning, so children can help it but ask for an explanation for everything that they cannot understand.

If you want to persuade someone, you can be able to do it by providing meaning to the information that is available to them and by linking what they are thinking with what you want them to think. To do this, you have to use the word "mean" as frequently as you need to during your conversation with the person whom you are trying to influence.

For example, when you are pitching an idea to a client, you can finish your presentation with lines such as "hiring me means you get the best services" or "using our services means fast results which means more money for you."

However, even without using the word "means," you can condition a person to associate certain ideas with certain feelings. This technique is often used in advertising to link products with positive experiences. For example, all Coca-Cola adverts showcase happy people doing exciting things because their marketing experts want you to believe that "Coca-Cola means happiness."

Using the Word "Because"

When you use the word "because" in a sentence, it indicates to the person you are talking to that "all questions have been answered," and they are more likely to give you what you want without bombarding you with lots of follow-up questions.

The word "because" starts almost all sentences that are used to answer the question "why?" So, when you preemptively use the word "because" in your statement, the person you are talking to will subconsciously feel as though all of his "why" questions have been addressed.

For example, when you ask your friend, "I need to borrow your car to go to the mall." He is more likely to have a follow-up question than if you had told him, "I need to borrow your car because I have to go to the mall." When he hears the first sentence, he will feel as though you haven't addressed your reason for borrowing his car. When he hears the second sentence, he will as if the latter part of the sentence (going to the mall) explains the former part of the sentence (borrowing the car).

Mind Control Techniques
What is Hypnosis?

If you ask the average person on the street what hypnosis is, they are more likely to come up with answers ranging from swinging pendulums to people doing crazy things such as barking like a dog. Not their fault. We've all been fed with terrible misconceptions regarding hypnosis by popular media. It is viewed as something increasingly weird or scary, almost as a form of black magic or some mumbo-jumbo.

In a purely scientific sense, hypnosis is related to different states of consciousness or awareness. We have a waking state or a state in which we are fully awake, alert and alive to real-world experiences. There is an awareness of what we experience in and around us. We move from different states of consciousness all through the day. For instance, you are enjoying a relaxing aroma massage treatment, and you begin to feel drowsy, your mind is roaming or subtly shifting from one state of consciousness into another.

Simply put, hypnosis is an altered state of awareness or being, which we move in and out of throughout the day. It occurs even when our eyes are wide open and can be induced without the use of words. For instance, you can be hypnotized simply by staring at a subject continuously. The most important aspect of hypnosis – it diminishes a person's ability to think rationally, evaluate information critically and make independent decisions.

Ever stared continuously at a fish tank? After staring for a while, your attention becomes absolutely focused, and you switch off or blank out from everything else happening in the surroundings. It is like nothing else apart from the fish tank, and you exist in the world. This is typically a hypnotic trance or altered state of mind or awareness. It draws your attention primarily on what is occurring internally than externally.

An important aspect of hypnosis and why it is popularly used by manipulators around the world is that reduces an individual's ability to think rationally. They become receptive to any information that is fed to them without applying much thought, irrespective of whether the idea is logical or not. This simply means that people in a trance state are susceptible to uncritically or unquestioning accept the notions/ideas that are fed to them. Their powers of logical analysis, rational decision making and objective judgments are completely eliminated.

This is precisely the level at which cult leaders lead their followers into doing exactly what they want in an absolutely unquestioning manner. When powers of judgment and decision making are reduced, people blindly follow what they've been led to believe.

Mind control hypnotism or hypnosis equips you with the arsenal to manipulate others.

What is Covert Hypnosis?

Covert hypnosis is when an attempt is made to communicate with the subject's unconscious mind without the subject knowing that he or she will be put through hypnosis. It comprises a string of technique such as conversational hypnosis or NLP (neuro-linguistic programming), body language and other powerful communication and interaction strategies.

The primary objective of covert hypnosis is to gradually change an individual's behavior at a subconscious level to lead the subject into believing that they changed their mind on their own accord. You simply lead them into believing that they weren't influencer or manipulated by changed their mind on their own.

When covert hypnosis is successfully performed, the subject isn't aware that he or she is being hypnotized. There is considerable debate about the fine line between conventional hypnotism and covert hypnotism. While standard hypnotism is about drawing the focus of the subject, covert hypnotism is primarily about relaxing the subject a bit or softening their stand by using deception, confusion, interruption and a series of other techniques.

If you've watched the series "The Mentalist," you'll realize that covert hypnosis is used in a particular instance when a perpetrator tries to influence various characters and tries to murder her employer.

8 Proven Covert Hypnosis Techniques

Here are some forms of covert hypnosis techniques for beginners

1. Deception

Deception is one of the most commonly practiced covert hypnosis techniques to lead the subject into doing what you want without them knowing about your real intentions. For instance, you may want a close friend to give up addiction and resort to plain deception to lead them away from their addiction triggers or suggest something false without making them catch your true intentions of making them give up alcohol or drugs.

As a practiced hypnotist, you create an illusion or sense of false reality to help the subject believe something you want them to. We have all been susceptible to deception at some point or the other. There is a tendency of believing fictional information without ever asking for details.

Clairvoyants, psychics, and hypnotists used this method generously to create an illusion by gaining the explicit trust of the subject through clever rapport-building techniques.

2. Eye Contact Clues

People almost always display a particular body language type that reflects their deepest thoughts and feelings. Hackneyed as it sounds, "Eyes are truly windows to one's soul." Analyzing an individual's body language (especially their eyes) will award you with a good sense of how a particular word, action, sound, image or emotion is perceived by him or her.

The subject is read based the direction's his or her eyes are darting in. Examine the subject's eyes thoroughly for cues. This technique is more complicated than it sounds and needs plenty of practice.

3. Misdirection

This covert hypnosis technique is widely used by magicians all over the world to manipulate their audience or create an illusion. Magicians sneakily use the power of misdirection to distract their audience's attention to another point of focus to perform a quick action that they wish to hide.

For instance, if you are attempting to get the subject to do something by directly sowing the suggestion, they are more consciously aware of your intentions. However, if you are accomplishing the same goal, you distract their attention elsewhere and make the same suggestion worded in another context.

4. Submodalities

There is great variance between the responses of different to the same information. This can be detected by the manipulator using several submodalities (under various contexts) to generate the desired response. Look for voice tone, body language, facial expressions and eyes cues. When the use of certain words or actions creates positive submodalities, you can continue using them to invoke specific feelings or emotions.

5. Generalized Reading

Generalized or warm reading is a covert hypnosis technique based on making a generalized observations or statements that could be applicable for just about anyone that do not take into account unique observations or responses gained from the subject.

Fortune tellers, psychic and clairvoyants use a lot of this technique to manipulate their clients into believing that the readings are unique to them, when in fact, these are general observations that can be applicable for just about any person.

For instance, "You are an ambitious person who also strives for happiness, contentment and inner peace. You've learned and evolved from your past experiences. You have overcome your past mistakes to look forward to new and exciting life ahead." You can ask any person to read this, and he or she will end up believing this was written only with him or her in mind. It leads the subject's mind to believe that it is about him or her since they are unique.

Warm readings can be used as icebreakers to establish a rapport of trust with the subject (by making seemingly accurate statements) before they begin to talk. This gives you the advantage to build upon the all too accurate beginning statement.

6. Hot Reading

Hot reading differs from general or warm readings in a manner that you have some prior information about the subject (which he or she is completely unaware of), which completely amazes them.

You've got to find a way to obtain important bits of information about a person without him or knowing about it, which can be tricky. The subject will then be led into believing that you have been blessed with supernatural or psychic abilities.

7. Cold Observations

While warm observations involve making generalized statements that can be applicable to everyone and hot observations are sneakily obtaining specific information about a person to use it to your advantage, cold observations are made based on your initial impression about a person by closely studying them. You then build upon the general statements by making more specific statements based on their responses.

It is regularly used by mentalists, psychics, and spiritualists to form an illusion that can accurately read a person's mind or perform telepathy. Subjects are led into believing that they are indeed everything they are told they are by the manipulator.

It comprises making vague statements after making a few first impression observations of an individual, which can easily be acquired after practicing a few people reading and analyzing skills. For example, you can simply say to your subject, "I have a feeling you are a self-assured and confident individual although you tend to hesitate at times based on past experiences." You wait for a response from the subject.

The subject can come up with a bunch of responses such as, "yes, you're right. I am generally confident and expressive but tend to be held back by past experiences" (which means they are generally confident people), "Oh yes, I do tend to reflect a lot on my past actions" (which means they are more shy and hesitant than self-assured and confident). Once they respond to a general statement, you can use their response to make more specific or direct statements about the person.

8. Ericksonian Hypnosis Theory

This technique comprises using stories, examples and anecdotes for eliminating the wall of resistance built by our subconscious mind. The hypnotizer or manipulator narrates a story, which ends with a moral that the manipulator desires to convey.

The subject's subconscious mind builds a connection or deep relationship with different aspects of the story. You lead the subject into emotionally linking with the story that sounds similar to the situation they are in currently.

This is s strategy for making indirect suggestions using a story to distract or divert the conscious mind, thus leaving the unconscious more receptive to suggestions.

Power-Packed Conversational Hypnosis Techniques

One form of covert hypnosis that can be used to manipulate someone into what you want is conversational hypnosis. It helps you establish an immediate connection with the other person so you can almost mind read them and lead them to do as you desire.

Among other things, conversational hypnosis gives you the ability to alter a person's state of consciousness right there and then, while driving them into a hypnotic trance. It will get people to obey what you are telling them to do without giving it a logical thought. Conversational hypnosis can be used as a tool for changing a person's behavior and getting them to act on your command. Here are a few time-tested secrets of conversational hypnosis unlocked.

1. Sharpen Your State of Awareness Recognition

To be an ace hypnotizer, you need to be fully aware of or identify trance signals in others. This becomes even more complex when the signals are subtle. Practice enhancing your state of consciousness or awareness so you can better recognize signals of other people changing states of awareness.

Once you gain expertise in the art of being aware of your state of consciousness, it will be easier to gain awareness of the slightest detail around you. Your senses will be open and receptive for quickly catching on to any changes you spot in the immediate environment.

2. Build on It

In this technique of conversational hypnosis, what you are actually doing is slowly sowing a seed of thought or idea in the mind of the other person, which you intend to keep growing over a period of time, one bit at a time.

It starts by asking the person to change something really tiny. Then build on that chain by requesting more and more change. Start with something simple and non-complicated during each session of hypnosis. To make them reach a gradual state of intense trace, gradually and progressively build upon the simple or easy request.

3. Controlling with the Voice

You have to have a distinct tone of voice for trance and nontrance states if you really wish to have a powerful effect on the mind of a person. During the entire hypnosis process, you must progressively move into your special trance tonality.

The idea is to clearly distinguish between your voices when the person transcends through different states of consciousness. Thus, the voice can be slightly lighter in a less intense state of trance and deeper when the trance state is more intense. This way you can control the movement of your subject from one state of consciousness to another simply by using your voice at will. They can be led to move from one state of awareness into another through the power of your voice alone.

4. Repetition

This is a form of controlling the mind through repeated exposure to a thought, idea or behavior pattern. Repetition is a covert hypnotic manipulation tactic used to expose your subject to the same idea or notion again and again until it is deeply embedded into their subconscious mind, and they start believing the notion to be true.

5. Compounding Effect

This technique simply means that each time your idea receives a positive response from the subject; you follow it up with a more powerful one. You are basically building on your last success point. When a suggestion works, you prim up the next one and have it ready for acceptance (greater odds of it being accepted if the earlier suggestion has been received positively).

In the event that your suggestion is met with a negative response, you start again from the last point of positive response and build on it.

6. Dramatic Words

'Hot words' is another brilliant conversational manipulation technique that is often used by glib conversationalists to hypnotize people. Our subconscious mind associates certain words and phrases with powerful emotions. There is a deep emotional or psychological significance linked to these words or phrases that almost always drives the subject into action.

Words such as "baby" "love" "trust" "assurance" and more incite a sense of warmth within the subject.

Once they respond to the hot words in a positive manner, you subtly begin to move to hypnotic words to first induce a state of relaxation, followed by a state of trance. For triggering a state of relaxation, you use words such as "relax." When you urge someone to relax, it triggers memories associated with relaxation such as lying on the beach or watching television. All the relaxation memories combine to make the person slip into a heightened state of relaxation.

This is followed by encouraging them to fixate their attention by using words such as "concentrate" or "focus." You have to emphasize on words that essentially convey that a person should pass their regular conscious state and do things more unconsciously. Words such as "spontaneous" invoke those reactions or responses.

7. Amplifying Words

Much like hot or hypnotic words that are spoken to generate a desired reaction through the process of hypnosis, amplifying words increase or accelerate its pace. When you want your subject to perform a specific action, use words like "right now", "instantly" "immediately", "suddenly" etc. They create a rather dramatic effect or tension and a more powerful effect on the subject's unconscious mind, thus leading them to a response.

Mind control involves using influence and persuasion to change the behaviors and beliefs in someone. That someone might be the person themselves or it might be someone else. Mind control has also been referred to as brainwashing, thought reform, coercive persuasion, mental control, and manipulation, just to name a few. Some people feel that everything is done by manipulation. But if that is true to be believed, then important points about manipulation will be lost. Influence is much better thought of as a mental continuum with two extremes. One side has influences that are respectful and ethical and work to improve the individual while showing respect for them and their basic human rights. The other side contains influences that are dark and destructive that work to remove basic human rights from a person, such as independence, the ability for rational thought, and sometimes their total identity.

When thinking of mind control, it is better to see it as a way to use influence on other people that will disrupt something in them, like their way of thinking or living. Influence works on the very basis of what makes people human, such as their behaviors, beliefs, and values. It can disrupt the very way they chose personal preferences or make critical decisions. Mind control is nothing more than using words and ideas to convince someone to say or do something they might never have thought of saying or doing on their own.

There are scientifically proven methods that can be used to influence other people. Mind control has nothing to do with fakery, ancient arts, or even magical powers. Real mind control really is the basis of a word that many people hate to hear. That word is marketing. Many people hate to hear that word because of the negative connotations associated with it. When people hear "marketing," they automatically assume that it refers to those ideas taught in business school. But the basis of marketing is not about deciding which part of the market to target or deciding which customers will likely buy this product. The basis of marketing is one very simple word. That word is "YES."

If a salesperson asks a regular customer to write a brief endorsement of the product they buy, hopefully, they will say yes. If someone asks their significant other to take some of the business cards to pass out at work, hopefully, they will say yes. If you write any kind of blog and ask another blogger to provide a link to yours on their blog, hopefully, they will say yes. When enough people say yes, the business or blog will begin to grow. With even more yesses, it will continue to grow and thrive. This is the very simple basis of marketing. Marketing is nothing more than using mind control to get other people to buy something or to do something beneficial for someone else. And the techniques can easily be learned.

The first technique in mind control is to tell people what you want them to want. Never tell people to think it over or take some time. That is a definite mind control killer. People already have too much going on in their minds. When they are told to think something over they will not. It will be forgotten, and then it will never happen. This has nothing to do with being stupid or lazy and everything to do with just being way too busy.

So the best strategy is to take the offensive and think for them. Everything must be explained in the beginning. Never assume that the other blogger will automatically understand the benefits of adding a link will be for them. Do not expect anyone to give a demonstration blindly. And merely asking for a testimonial, while it might garner an appositive response, probably will not garner a well-formed testimonial to the product. Instead, be prepared to explain the blog, show examples, and offer compelling reasons why this merger will be a benefit to both parties. Have the demonstration laid out in great detail with notes on what to say when and visuals to go along with the notes, so all the other person has to do is present the information. Offer the customer a few variations of testimonials that have already been received and ask them to choose one and personalize it a bit. Always be specific in explaining what is desired. Explain why it is desired. Show how this will work. Tell the person how to do it and why they should do it. If done correctly it will feel exactly like one friend advising another friend on which is the best path to take. And the answer will be yes simply because saying yes makes so much sense.

Think of the avalanche. Think of climbing all the way to the top of the highest mountain ever. Now, at the top, think of searching for the biggest heaviest boulder that exists on the mountain. Now, picture summoning up superhuman strength to push this boulder, dislodging it from the place it has rested for years and years. Once this boulder is loosened, it rolls easily over the edge of the cliff, crashing into thousands of other boulders on its way down the mountain, taking half of the mountain with it in a beautiful cascade of rocks and dirt. Imagine sitting there smiling cheerfully at the avalanche that was just created.

Marketing and mind control are very like creating an avalanche. Getting the first person to answer yes might be difficult. But each subsequent yes will be easier and easier. And always start at the top, never the bottom. Starting at the top is definitely more difficult, and it is more likely to come with more negative responses than positive responses in the beginning. But starting at the top also yields a much greater reward when the avalanche does begin. And the results will be far greater than beginning at the bottom of the mountain. Yes, the small rock is easier to push over. Then it can be built upon by pushing over another small rock, then another. This way can work, but it will take much longer than being successful at the top. No one ever went fishing for the smallest fish in the pond or auditioned for the secondary role just to be safe. Everyone wants that top prize. Do not be afraid to go for it.

On the other hand, never ask for the whole boulder the first time. Ask for part of it. This may seem directly contradictory but it is not. Always start with a small piece. Make the beginning easier for everyone to see. Let other people use their own insight to see the end result. When the first bit goes well, then gradually ask for more and more and more.

Think of writing a guest spot for someone else who has their own blog. By sending in the entire manuscript first, there is a greater risk of rejection. Begin small. Send them a paragraph or two discussing them the idea. Then make an outline of the idea and send that in an email. Then write the complete draft you would like them too use and send it along. When asking a customer for a testimonial, start by asking for a few lines in an email. Then ask the customer to expand those few lines into a testimonial that covers at least half a typed page. Soon the customer will be ready for an hour-long webcast extolling the virtues of the product and your great customer service skills.

Everything must have a deadline that really exists. The important word here is the word 'real'. Everyone has heard the salesperson who said to decide quickly because the deal might not be available later or another customer was coming in and they might get it. That is a total fabrication and everyone knows it to be true. There are no impending other customers and the deal is not going to disappear. There is no real sense of urgency involved. But everyone does it. There are too many situations where people are given a totally fake deadline by someone who thinks it will instill a great sense of urgency for completion of the task. It is not only totally not effective but completely unneeded. It is a simple matter to create true urgency. Only leave free things available for a finite amount of time. When asking customers for testimonials be certain to mention the last possible day for it to be received to be able to be used. Some people will be unable to assist, but having people unable to participate is better than never being able to begin.

Always give before you receive. And do not ever think that giving is fifty-fifty. Always give much more than is expected in return. Before asking for a testimonial from a satisfied customer, be sure to make numerous acts of exceptional customer service. Before asking a blog writer for a link, link theirs to yours many times. This is not about helping someone out so they will help you. This is all about being so totally generous that the person who is asked for the favor cannot possibly say no. It might mean extra work, but that is how to influence other people.

Always stand up for something that is much bigger than average. Do not just write another blog on how to do something. Use an important issue to take a stand and defend the stance with unbeatable logic and fervent passion. Do not just write a how-to manual. Choose a particular idea and sell people on it, using examples of other people with the same idea living the philosophy.

Never feel shame. This does not mean being extremely extroverted to the point of silliness or having a total lack of conscience in business dealings. In the case of mind control shamelessness refers to a total complete belief that this course of action is the best possible course and everyone will benefit greatly from it. This is about writing the best possible blog ever and believing that everyone needs to read it to be able to improve their lives. It is about believing in a particular product so deeply that the feeling is that everyone will benefit from using it. It is knowing deep inside that this belief is the most correct belief ever and everyone should believe it.

Mind control uses the idea that someone's decisions and emotions can be controlled using psychological means. It is using powers of negotiation or mental influence to ensure the outcome of the interaction is more favorable to one person over the other. This is basically what marketing is: convincing someone to do something particular or buy something in particular. Being able to control someone else's mind merely means understanding the power of human emotion and being able to play upon those emotions. It is easier to have a mental impact on people if there is a basic understanding of human emotions. Angry people will back down when the subject of their anger is not afraid. Angry people feed upon the fear of others. Guilt is another great motivator. Making someone feel guilty for not thinking or feeling, in the same manner, is a wonderful way to get them to give in. Another way to use mind control over someone is to point out how valuable they are to the situation.

Emotional Manipulation

Everyone sometime in their life will have felt the cold grasp of an emotional manipulator coming inside to a piece of them which they feel incapable to safeguard regardless of how hard they attempt.

The point of a manipulator is to do only that, manipulation! The point of their game is to deal with the individual who is their picked injured individual; the purpose behind this is if they deal with the other, at that point that individual can be made from multiple points of view flexible to the manipulators wants, along these lines decreasing any type of risk to the manipulator Usually however, it is simply the manipulator neurosis and low regard which goes crazy in their mind giving them the feeling that anyone and everyone is, or could be a danger.

To conquer this and to protect themselves as far as they could tell; they will attempt to fool the picked injured individual into feeling helpless, so whether the unfortunate casualty was to assault, they would ordinarily be not able.

There are four fundamental kinds of manipulator to watch out for, and these are:

The Rejecter

This manipulator is an especially terrible one and is slicing directly profoundly of the most profound fear of 95% of mankind which is that of being distant from everyone else. This fear is destroying to such an extent that individuals will do pretty much anything to stay away from it, including attempting to win the manipulators warmth.

The Insulter

This kind of manipulator is "the joyful one" ceaselessly splitting the odd joke to a great extent, remarks about weight gain/misfortune, hair loss and whatever other territory that the unfortunate casualty feels hesitant about, however then when the injured individual says how they feel, the manipulator returns with "I'm just joking" or "don't get so stirred up" (an attempt at manslaughter assault).

The Intimidator

This style is increasingly noticeable, yet they will likewise attempt to keep it inconspicuous. This style of manipulation works by unobtrusive or prominent changes in the non-verbal communication, heavier breathing, showing outrage, dismissing, raised voice or an appearance of they are prepared to assault. A change made regularly enough utilizing a similar example yet without knowing why, might frequently leave an injured individual confounded and nervous fearing the beginning of physical viciousness.

The Decent Person

This manipulator is by a wide margin one of the most underhanded. Acting like a companion and giving the feeling that they are on the exploited people side, gradually gain their trust and readiness to open up the heart and afterward inconspicuously drop in the debasing remarks and how in spite of the fact that the unfortunate casualty is an incredible companion a portion of their perspectives and interests simply are wrong and afterward the manipulator will seal the assault with, I'm just letting you know since I give it a second thought, giving the injured individual the appearance someone to feel upheld by and go to when out of luck, yet in all embodiment making them subordinate.

Manipulator are once in a while the very in the face types (physical viciousness) however the most unsafe; are the enthusiastic sorts who get inside their unfortunate casualty's mind, commandeering their feelings leaving them befuddled and helpless, giving the manipulator all the power. In the event that you feel awkward around someone however don't have the foggiest idea why, the odds are you are in their grasp and much of the time the two gatherings are absolutely unconscious, yet it is your obligation to stop the game.

Subliminal Manipulation

As a matter of fact, mind control can be as simple as subliminal suggestion used to steer one in the direction you want rather than the direction they were going autonomously.

There are many schools of thought in regards to mind control, but for this book, let's look at a common example of mind control to start. Color, smell, sight, sound, and taste are used on the consumer by every company selling a product to advance their customers and sales. When you enter your local grocery store, often there are fresh cut flowers at the entrance. Now, how often have you bought those flowers? Chances are, never, if maybe a time or two because you forgot a special occasion. Grocers use the presence of these flowers as a means of manipulating the subconscious of their customers. Fresh cut flowers are, well, fresh. Ripe. Pleasant. They subliminally convey they thought of freshness, and your local grocery store wants you to be thinking about all the fresh produce they have waiting for you. More often, these grocers make more on the sale of their fresh produce over name brand canned and frozen produce, and if you buy the produce they have available, more of your dollars go in their pocket as opposed to mass production companies.

Every day, you are exposed to one form of mind control or another. Product placement on television and in movies. The music you hear in a store or even an elevator. Friends that are so convincing, you can't help but agree, or you find yourself always saying yes to them.

Re-education is a very optimal, but controversial tool in mind control. The ability to re-educate another person's previous thought process or beliefs is possible, but can take time. At the heart of re-education sits repetition. I repeat, repetition. By repeating the same belief, idea, or thought to another person, repeatedly, you are impressing upon them the change from their own ideas towards your own. And this repetition leads to immersion in the idea or action you want them to follow. Being immersed in an idea, the idea in question always being repeated, the idea or goal always being spoken of, leads to the individual re-examining their previous feelings about the issue. Re-examining one's feelings often leads to them coming to a new conclusion. Your conclusion. You have just exerted a form of mind control on another individual, and now they agree with you.

Priming an individual is another effective way to get what you want. Some who see this activity negatively may refer to in as indoctrination, but the goal is not to necessarily start a cult. You are just trying to get others to agree with you, and are trying to use all the available tools you possess to your advantage. Priming involves softening a person towards you and your ideas, easing them into the thought that you know what is best. Softening can include hours of conversation, empathizing with them and showing them that you care or love them. You care about what happens, you understand them. Once you have a foundation of trust through understanding and priming, soft persuasion towards the new idea, belief, or action can be introduced. It is imperative that you have formed a mutual bond or respect with the person who you want to influence. And it is a given that change takes time.

A few techniques to help you on your path to persuasion using coercion may involve thinking for others, being specific in your logic and requests, creating a real sense of urgency, and stressing the importance of your goal or idea. When presenting someone with a change in long held ideas or requests, thinking for them takes the pressure of deciding off them. People often have enough on their mental plates as it is, you shouldn't be asking them to take on more, especially when you can do the heavy lifting for them. Explain exactly why they should see things your way, offering as many examples as possible as to the correctness to your idea, proof that what you want is not only right, but it is proven to be effective or accurate. Once you have specifically lined out why they should agree with you, tell them what is next and why things need to be done your way. Be friendly but as firm and confident in your pitch to them as you need be, and often discouraging questions until you are finished explaining your stance helps steer others in your direction. They often forget their questions or objections as they listen to you explain what you want, why, and what you think needs to happen next to achieve the goal. It is all about the goal.

While we are on the subject of your goals and what you want to achieve, it is imperative to stress the importance of what you want to achieve. If others are consistently being spoken with on how important the idea or goal is, and specifics on why it is so important, eventually they start to see your idea as more than just something you want, but an issue of utmost importance. Your thought or goal becomes something more, and it should be more to you too. it should be a movement. A goal doesn't have to be a social ideal to be a movement, you just need others to feel it's importance as much as you do. Everyone wants to be on the right side of history, no matter how big or small the issue is. And all it takes is someone to see your want as a matter that needs to be addressed or adjusted, and where there is one person who agrees with you, there are two, and more soon to follow.

So, your idea, goal, or thought is now more than just something you want. Other people want it too. And it is not just important, it is imperative. And it needs to happen now. Creating a sense of urgency is another effective form of utilizing mind control techniques to your benefit. Making urgent statements, or claiming that this situation is time sensitive will create an emotional response in those you wish to influence or persuade. A specific deadline needs to be in place, but the idea that this can't wait long needs to be an underlying sentiment. The quicker you get other people on board, the more important you convince them your want is, the more urgent they believe things are, the less resistance you will run into. The more information backing your idea or goal people are given, the more likely they will let you think for them and just go with the flow. The more urgent the matter is, the less time people have to ask discouraging questions or second guess their shift in ideas.

Being consistent is the most important aspect of implementing mind control techniques to get what you want. Consistently repeating what you want, and be consistent when rejecting old ideas or goals. Be consistent when speaking about what needs to happen, when and why. These factors should be underlined, in bold print, repeated regularly, and the time sensitivity need to be stressed.

There is nothing wrong with being a little pushy to get what you want out of your life. Another great technique when using mind control is to ask small things of others, or asking for small changes in another's ideas, and then expanding from there. Let's use a raise from your employer as an example. If you want a decent increase in pay, don't ask for your top dollar pay increase. Ask for a small increase in pay based on your performance and loyalty. Your boss will agree (considering you are worthy of the raise to begin with) and think that they got off cheap keeping you happy. After you have reached the first step in reaching your ultimate pay goal, ask for more work. Let your employer know you are more than happy taking on more responsibility. You can possibly save them money if you are doing more work than before, they may not have to hire another employee to work weekends if you are willing to come in for a few hours on a Saturday. Now, you have a pay increase, but you have more responsibility. It only seems fair that you are paid a little more now that you are a more valuable resource for your employer to utilize. It's better they give you another slight pay increase to cover your knowledge and expertise in the workplace than bother trying to hire another employee to replace you. You see how simple it can be? Now, that isn't saying that you have a boss or employer this would work on, but if you are implementing the other tools you have in your fast-growing arsenal, you are now a very well-liked employee and co-worker who knows how to influence and persuade others to see things the way you do. Your employer may not like the idea of paying you even more than before, but sometimes it's not just your work ethic that matters, sometimes it's what you bring to the table for everyone you encounter.

It is not easy to say no to someone who you feel a debt to. The final technique of mood control we should consider is generosity. You should always strive to give more than you take from others. When you give more of your time, your effort, your attention, to others, they appreciate it. They remember it. And, when the time comes that you want something in return, it is much harder to say no, or disagree, or refuse to cooperate with another who has freely offered up so much to them. Even in circumstances or changes others may not want to agree or get on board with, if they know that you have been offered the same courtesy by you previously, they find it hard to go against you. It falls back to persuasion, influence, and reciprocation. Most often, those that you have committed your time and attention to will return the favor. Even if you are met with resistance by someone who you have given to, a gentle reminder of what you have done for them is often all that is needed to get them on board with what you want. Sometimes it isn't the loudest voice in the room that matters, but the most consistent and softest from the individual who has done the most to help others. That soft but firm voice can be yours, you only need to take your opportunities as they present themselves.

The Art of Persuasion

Power and control over other people

Strong individuals appear to have the option to identify with a truth - rationally tough individuals don't give away their power.

It's something we all do in some cases. Perhaps you let your associate's awful mind-set ruin your day. Or on the other hand maybe you let somebody's analysis of you harm your self-esteem.

Whenever you enable somebody to have a negative impact over the manner in which you think, feel, or act, you give them control over your life. It will deny you of the psychological quality you need to have to arrive at your most prominent potential.

Sometimes, it's undeniable when you surrender your power. Losing your cool and doing something you later regret is a prime example.

But on the other hand it's conceivable to surrender your power in progressively unperceivable ways. You probably won't understand you're doing it.

The need to control others may not sound good to you. In case you have an inclination toward understanding an individual, you'd never want to control another person.

In any case, controllers are out there. They need to micromanage what you say, how you act, even what you think discreetly as far as you could tell. It could be your boss, your mate, or even your parent. You can't act naturally around them. They demand being your top requirement and need undue impact over your life. They may push your buttons to get a passionate response out of you since they need to misuse it as a shortcoming. They have no regard for you or your limits.

There are a lot of speculations why somebody would need to control you. One is that individuals who can't control themselves start controlling others. This occurs on an enthusiastic level. An individual loaded with instabilities needs to create a constructive feeling of self from other individuals, on the grounds that their confidence is too low to even consider doing it for themselves.

Perhaps individuals control since they fear being deserted. They don't have a sense of safety in their connections and are frequently trying to check whether they're going to be double-crossed. The oddity is that their conduct makes precisely what they fear the most happen.

Maybe these individuals are narcissists hoping to control their condition using any and all means. This would mean other individuals are pawns. They're helpful apparatuses in the narcissist's reality to be utilized as the individual pleases. It's not very kind — to them you're just a decent pawn. The issue with this point of view is that these controlling harassers frequently makes us wonder, "Why me? Why do I feel like an object?"

The easiest explanation is that you're a decent, commendable individual. There's nothing amiss with you. You don't have an ulterior motive, and you don't deserve to be slighted. It might seem like an extreme idea, yet what the controller needs is the thing that you have:

You're ready to like yourself, reliably and without consistent updates from the outside world- you know that you're commendable.

You're secure in your achievements, your status, and your general place throughout everyday life.

Your consideration makes other individuals feel better.

You can support and celebrate other individuals' success — you're not scared by others' favorable luck.

Given each one of those things, you realize you have earned positive regards, however a controlling individual is too scared to even consider giving it to you. They believe they should pare you down. It's the only way they can endure being around you.

While there is a clarification for why the controller is how they are, it doesn't make a difference. It's an ideal opportunity to recover your power and spotlight individual needs. This means defining immovable limits and shielding the controller from venturing forth on the opposite side of them. Choose what you're never again ready to forfeit. A few models include:

Never again be made to feel like your thoughts and commitments don't make a difference.

Not giving them a chance to depreciate your achievements and speak condescendingly to you.

Not enabling anybody to push your buttons.

Not willing to repress your own requirements for this individual.

The controller has been the recipient of your positive attitude for a really long time. This is an ideal opportunity to place that back in your own corner. It's about self-safeguarding, and you'll realize when you're doing it right since you won't feel like an object any longer. Truth be told, the controller presumably won't have much use for you.

Make it flawlessly obvious to yourself every day that you're in the driver's seat and you're not searching for any other individual to fill that position.

Here are a few different ways you may give away your own power without acknowledging it:

1. You yield to remorseful fits.

If you change your conduct if somebody pulls at your heartstrings, you give that individual control over you. Shout out, adhere to your promise, and don't give in in spite of when somebody attempts to play on your feelings.

2. You permit another person's assessment of you to affect your self-esteem.

Some people won't care for you and some people won't care for your decisions. You don't need to give their assessments a chance to influence how you feel about yourself, in any case. Feeling terrible about yourself dependent on what somebody says or how that individual feels about you gives that individual an excess of control over you.

3. You don't set up sound limits.

You choose who to permit into your life. If you become angry at individuals who take up a lot of your vitality, it's a sign you aren't defining clear limits. Set up clear physical, passionate, and money related limits.

4. You whine pretty much about every one of the things you need to do.

You additionally get the chance to choose how to manage your time. You aren't compelled to get down to business, see the specialist, or go to a family gathering. There will be results if you don't do those things, however they're still decisions.

5. You hold feelings of resentment.

Resentment won't reduce the other individual's place in your life; however, it can unleash ruin in yours without outside influence.

Reliving outrage from the past enables a person to consume space in your life. This isn't to imply that you have to permit lethal individuals into your life- - you shouldn't. Simply don't squander your psychological assets on them.

6. You change your objectives since you were rejected.

Surrendering in the wake of being rejected enables a person to figure out what you'll do with your life. Regardless of whether you got denied for a promotion or turned down for a group road trip, don't surrender. Just because other individuals don't perceive your potential doesn't mean you will fail.

7. You set out to refute somebody.

When somebody questions you, it very well may entice you to decide to refute them. Ensure your motivation is about your craving to succeed, not tied in with persuading individuals that you're more significant than they gave you credit for.

8. You let other individuals draw out the most terrible aspects of you.

You're going to keep running into individuals who can draw out the most noticeably terrible thing in you. These people may incite you to make statements you regret or make you do things you wouldn't regularly do. Remain consistent with your qualities and decline to give others a chance to have a negative impact over you.

9. You put time into discussing individuals that you don't care for.

Every time you spend effort contemplating somebody you don't care for, or whining about somebody you would prefer not to be near, is 60 additional seconds you give that individual. Harping on antagonistic individuals permits them to have control over your soul.

10. You strive to keep away from analysis.

Criticism from others can be instrumental in helping you be your best. If you esteem other individuals' information to an extreme, in any case, you may abstain from doing whatever could prompt analysis. It's difficult to carry on with your best life when you're focused on satisfying individuals.

Step by step instructions to take back your power

If you see that you're giving your power endlessly, you're not the only one. Everybody does it sometimes. The uplifting news is, it's never past the point where it is impossible to begin reclaiming your power.

Focus on turning into the driver - as opposed to the traveler - in your life. Try to remain responsible for how you think, feel, and act and you'll help construct the psychological muscle you need to have to arrive at your most noteworthy potential.

Methods of Persuasion

Appeals to reason

Reason should be the backbone behind every single successful conversation. As this book is to a great extent about basic deduction, a great part of the book's substance will show the reader how to utilize sound and substantial thinking, while at the same time maintaining a strategic distance from the false notions and other manipulative endeavors used to convince others.

Appeals to emotion

Be aware that people are not always completely balanced creatures, and there is nothing amiss with conceding that we help other people since we are driven by sympathy, not rational or valid justifications of conventional contentions. Also, we frequently react considerably more to enthusiastic interests, so creating proper and reasonable approaches to speak about our expectations, fears, joys, bitterness, etc… can positively upgrade the chances of effectively convincing others.

Claims to the speaker's very own believability, dependability and character.

Significantly more so when convincing with a composed speech, crowds judge the source (the speaker). Truth be told, if crowds don't have confidence in a speaker or see that the speaker isn't really educated, at that point the influence regularly flops before it's even genuinely tuned in to or analyzed fundamentally.

Accordingly, speakers must do a ton of work to show to crowds that they are educated and energetic about the subject (it's ideal to do as such in the presentation), and they should exhibit that the substance of the speech is being conveyed for the group of spectators' advantage. This is done both with content and with conveyance.

Speakers ought to plainly disclose to the crowd why they are specialists. At that point, show that skill with a certain, rehearsed, smooth conveyance. Reading eliminates one's believability; faltering too much, utilizing an excessive number of verbal influences, (for example, "um," "ah" or "like") likewise hurts a speaker's validity.

In a perfect world, speakers would find a proper blend of these three strategies for influence to develop a convincing contention.

Influential history and background

The power and pervasiveness of influence have prompted a lot of logical research examining the variables that make an influential intrigue viable. During the 1950s, Carl Hovland and his partners at Yale University led the main investigation of influence in what was known as the Yale Communication Project. The Yale gathering confirmed that four components are available in all influence settings:

- A source who conveys the influential message.

- The message itself.

- An objective individual or group of spectators who gets the message (beneficiary).

- Some setting wherein the message is received.

After receiving data dealing with influence, the scientists suggested that for a powerful intrigue to work, the message beneficiary must focus on, appreciate, learn, acknowledge, and hold the message and its decision in memory. Individuals' level of commitment in this way was believed to be controlled by different qualities of the source, message, beneficiary, and powerful setting. For instance, a profoundly mind boggling message may be too hard to even think about comprehending and in this way, unfit to be learned, acknowledged, or held.

Later research appeared, that influence regularly doesn't rely upon the particular contentions in a message that individuals learn and recollect- rather, on what remarkable intellectual (mental) responses they have in light of those contentions. That is, the thing that matters most when individuals are effectively handling the message isn't realizing what is in the message, however people's opinion of the message.

As indicated by this psychological reaction approach, influence is more probable when the beneficiary has positive convictions toward the message and more uncertain when the beneficiary's considerations about the message are troublesome. For instance, two people may both become familiar with similar subtleties of a proposition to expand the interstate speed limit but then have uncontrollably various musings (e.g., "I'll have the option to get to work quicker" versus "It will make driving even more hazardous").

Current theories of persuasion

The educational and psychological ways to deal with influence concentrated on change of frame of mind through dynamic, effortful reasoning. Nonetheless, study has likewise demonstrated that occasionally individuals are convinced to change their frames of mind when they are not pondering the data in the message.

Rather, they base their actions on straightforward, affiliated, or heuristic procedures that require less subjective exertion. Joining these various thoughts, Richard Petty and John Cacioppo's elaboration probability model (ELM) and Shelly Chaiken's heuristic-orderly model (HSM) are two comparable hypotheses presented during the 1980s that recommend that both effortful and non-effortful procedures can deliver disposition change in various circumstances.

As indicated by these models, when individuals are inspired and ready to assess all the data applicable to the message's position (high elaboration), they will pursue the focal or methodical course to influence. This is similar to the psychological reaction approach, whereby individuals' good or ominous musings about the message and their trust in them decide the level of change in their frame of mind.

Interestingly, when individuals are not pondering the benefits of the message (low elaboration), they can now be impacted by procedures requiring less subjective exertion. For instance, individuals can depend on alternate ways (e.g., "The package is great—it must be a decent toothpaste.") to choose when they concur with or like something. In these cases, individuals are said to take the fringe or heuristic course to influence.

For this situation, the models guarantee that people will utilize the focal (orderly) course when they are both propelled and ready to consider the substance of the message keenly. If in any way, shape or form, they are reluctant or unfit to participate in effortful reasoning, they will pursue the fringe (heuristic) course to influence.

Research utilizing the data and psychological reaction methodologies recognized various source, message, beneficiary, and logical factors that influenced the decisions. Incidentally, it was uncertain from those examinations precisely when and how every factor would influence frame of mind change. For instance, in certain studies a profoundly tenable source upgraded influence, yet in others the source repressed influence.

Be that as it may, the two distinct courses to influence illustrated in the ELM and HSM give a profitable system to decide when and how these factors will prompt a change in mindset. Specifically, the ELM holds that any factor inside the influence setting may assume one of a few roles. To begin with, when individuals are not considering the message, the variable is handled as a straightforward sign that impacts dispositions by simple affiliation or heuristic procedures.

Second, when individuals are altogether thinking about the benefits of the message, the variable will be investigated as a contention, predisposition continuously preparing the message, or influenced by trust in the contemplations created.

At last, when believing isn't compelled to be high or low by different components, the variable may be influenced by how much preparation is involved as an indicator of whether it merits placing exertion into assessing the message. The various roles for factors as clarified by the ELM give the premise as to how remarkably source, message, beneficiary, and setting elements influence decision making.

Source variables in persuasion

The source is the individual or substance who conveys the enticing intrigue, and various source qualities have been shown to impact disposition change. Two of the most commonly examined source factors are believability and engaging quality. Believability alludes to the source's (a) aptitude and (b) dependability. A specialist source is one who has applicable information or experience in regard to the theme of the enticing message. A reliable source is one who needs ulterior thought processes and communicates fair suppositions dependent on the data as the person in question sees it.

You may think about a doctor (master) and your closest companion (reliable) to be sound sources. Engaging quality alludes to how physically or socially engaging and affable the source is. For instance, TV commercials regularly use runway models and captivating famous people to get individuals to like their items. By and large (yet not constantly), trustworthy and alluring sources are more powerful than unpleasant sources.

Predictable with the ELM's various jobs theory, source factors have been shown to impact influence in a few unique ways in various circumstances. Consider, for instance, a commercial for a brand of cleanser that shows an alluring individual utilizing the item. Individuals frequently partner allure with positive sentiments, and under low elaboration conditions, when there is minimal effortful made pondering the message, they may conclude that they like the cleanser basically in light of the fact that the source makes them feel better.

Under high elaboration conditions, when believing is broad, individuals may analyze the beauty of the speaker as proof that the item gives them excellent hair. Even further, they may have more trust in the musings they have if they feel that the spokesperson recognizes and understands what they are discussing in depth.

What's more, if individuals don't know the extent to which they should think about the message, the magnificence of the source may instigate them to give more consideration to the commercial and its message. This would build influence if what the source says is convincing- however if the message isn't convincing, thinking increasingly about it could prompt less influence. Other source factors influence by similar components.

Self-Manipulation

Are you happy when people believe what you say? If you are, then you'll be happy to hear there's a way of achieving this effect systematically, through the cultivation of understanding the non-verbal, physical cues which form your perceptions of other people and vice versa. Are you happy when people stop what they're doing to pay attention to what you have to say? Obviously, it is a sign they think you're worth listening to. That's why judges and House Speakers use the gavel to call for silence and attention. Sometimes people are distracted, fidgety and unwilling to collect themselves long enough to listen (particularly politicians trying to get re-elected seated in legislative chambers).

All these factors add up to whether communication is effective or not. You're not the Speaker of the House. You have no gavel. So it's important that you're able to communicate effectively. Slamming things on the table might get people's attention, but that's not the type of attention you're looking for. You need to send the message that you are worth listening to. People who are worth listening to convey a certain sense of self which is rooted in confidence. That message is sent via all the verbal and non-verbal clues we give others. Our understanding of where our weaknesses and strengths lie can inform a better understanding of those same qualities in others.

Authority and Influence

Authority and influence are two entirely different things. To be honest, I'd rather be in a position of influence that one of authority. Influence is subtle. Authority is obvious. Influence is covert. Authority is overt. As an influencer, you have much more latitude then you might in a position of authority, because people in positions of authority are bound by the conventions of that same authority. For instance, a government leader may want to enact legislation, but is unable to, due to a fractious legislative body. But lobby groups, citizens' groups and non-governmental organizations can wield great influence in moving that fractious legislative body and getting the job done. Authority does a good job of looking powerful, but influence is the little man behind the curtain, actually getting things done.

To wield influence, it's not necessary to be in a position of authority or power for this reason. Influence is like the water that eventually erodes stone – subtle and unseen, but very real. While authority may well be the Hulk. Influence is the Ninja, stalking its objectives with determination, consistency and persistent dedication. Influential skill is a very desirable aptitude to cultivate for this reason.

The Center for Creative Leadership has established that influence has three essential components and an accompanying set of tactics: emotion, logic and cooperation. The first of these is probably the most accessible road to influence, as people's emotional lives are very close to the surface, most of the time. Appealing to the those you want to enlist to your cause via their emotions involves expressing your own conviction about whatever that cause is and moreover, expressing a belief that they have a pivotal part to play in the realization of your vision.

To make an effective emotional appeal, your powers of communicative interpretation come to the forefront. Who are you appealing to? Knowing this is key to effectively mounting an appeal rooted in emotion. What are the person's values and beliefs? What goals is this person shooting for and how can you help them get there? How does your vision uphold all these emotional factors and honor them? Being keenly aware of the values of the person you're talking to and how you can weave those values into your vision is how you build support using an influential emotional appeal.

Appealing to someone's logic involves showcasing the benefits of your vision to the organization or group and also, the person you're appealing to. A strong case built on logic will be accompanied by concrete evidence that your cause is not only viable, but desirable, in terms of implementation. This tactical style of influence demands that you be intimately connected with the nuts and bolts of your vision and passionate about influencing others to support it. Be fully prepared to defend your vision against objections by reading your plan, or idea through the eyes of a critic. Your critical deconstruction of your vision is a crucial part of the success of a logical appeal.

Positive team-building can result from a well-crafted cooperative appeal, in which you outline a plan or project in terms of mutual support and benefit. Creating a consultative framework for all parties to involve themselves in implementation is highly effective as a way of building influence. As you put people to work, you display confidence in their abilities. This creates strong networks of influence, as people don't forget those who've given them opportunities. They also don't forget strong leadership that results in effective action. By applying a cooperative appeal in support of a vision or project, you're not only realizing your goal, but you're undergirding your influence. From the process, it's inevitable that you will also grow new thought leaders for your organization, which is nothing but positive and casts you as a visionary.

Effective influence combines all three strategies concurrently and builds organizational confidence in your abilities. Where authority can prescribe, influence can actually fill the prescription. The doctor may pull down the big bucks, but the pharmacist delivers the cure.

So wielding influence is about building networks, knowing who you're talking to and being capable of providing logical and compelling reasons for what you have in mind. In learning to build your influential power, you're engaging your powers of communicative interpretation, emotional intelligence and critical thinking. All these factors, in the practice of influence, are hallmarks of leadership. In developing these skills, you're becoming a more well-rounded person and a force to be reckoned with.

Modelling Excellence

Influence is also inherent in your actions, your demeanor and your treatment of other people. Your work habits, your attention to detail, your presentation and your likeability all work together. They make you someone who is capable of wielding influence in any situation or organization. All these factors are just as important as your messaging, your knowledge and training and your people-reading skills.

People want to work with those they like. They want to spend their (at least) eight hours per day, five days per week, around people they find easy to get along with, helpful and cooperative. That's the bare minimum. If you're hoping to develop your influence in the workplace, then it goes without saying that you need to go the extra mile when it comes to modelling excellence.

Excellent employees don't just come in to work on time and leave a little late. They're not just willing to help and cooperate. Excellent employees see details others don't. They tie up loose ends, volunteer for projects others aren't necessarily interested in and help to create an environment of harmonious efficiency and genial collegiality. These are the foundations of excellence. Out of that foundation grows the solid stuff of organizational integrity, built by quality work that is doing a lot more than collecting a pay check. It's building something as part of a team and intentionally so.

How excellence is modelled is in the details many overlook. Excellent employees sweat that (apparently) small stuff, because they know it matters. Excellence is a collection of minutia that culminates in a whole. Your mood in the workplace. Your reputation among your peers. The quality of your work. The quality of your interactions. Your place on the team. Your consistency and commitment. These are all components of excellence and they're worthy of emulation. That's why others will emulate it. Those who aren't interested in doing so – who watch with jaded, envious eyes as excellence builds its influential power - are of no consequence. They're not interested and that won't go unnoticed when push comes to shove, or downsizing comes to town. What matters is that you're being the change you want to see. Modelling excellence means making yourself an icon of your vision and its soundness. This is what gets you heard, noticed and influencing those around you.

Client care excellence

You are likely to retain clients who feel you understand them even when they aren't particularly communicative, verbally. It is a sign they feel that you have internalized their needs, when, with just a gesture or two, they can let you know where they're at. This also fosters a sense of familiarity and collegiality that inspires customer loyalty. They will feel that you value them, because it's clear you can read them well. In short, by being able to perceive your clients' non-verbal communication, you endear yourself to them and make of yourself a trusted friend. Likewise, you need to be understood by them without either party having to resort to long emails or sitting through endless, time-wasting meetings. Solid business relationships are all about ease of communication and communal satisfaction with their quality. Being able to read the non-verbal cues offered by your clients can set you apart as an intuitive, savvy leader.

When excellence is inherent in your work and communications style, it will typify your client relationships. This is undeniable. The same excellence you model in your day to day work flows into the client relationship, strengthening it and sustaining it in a world of competitive challengers. Client care is what sets the best apart. As always, God is in the details. Understanding client need is rooted in understanding the client, the rhythms of the business involved, branding, budgeting and human resources. All of this information is your business and having a strong command of it, as well as an open and communicative relationship with your clients, can set you well apart. You are there when needed and you are effective. Excellent custom care amounts to a sense of service, a word too seldom heard. It should be your very favorite word when it comes to your clients, even if those clients who are internal (your co-workers).

Some minor factors to consider which may sometimes elude us amount to social niceties that also count as body language. These are forms of communication that continue to be important, regardless of their diminished cultural significance in some circles. It's important to understand the following information about engagement in the course of business interactions. These are professional interactions, not personal ones. For that reason, please read the following as a proviso against entirely preventable faux pas. Little slips in such seemingly inconsequential areas may seem excusable, but they can cost you valuable influence that you're trying to build up, not tear down. They matter.

Firm handshake

Have you ever thought about what a firm handshake says to your current or potential client? A firm, confident handshake sends the message that you're resolved and in control. Even today, the message of a firm handshake is that of competence and reliability. It means business, in the most basic sense. There was a day, not so very long ago, when women in business (who were rare), didn't extend their hands to be shaken by male business people. Women simply operated on a different level than men did in those times. These days, though, women are expected to similarly deliver a strong, confident handshake, which does not linger unduly, but is not retracted suddenly, as though being snatched from a fiery furnace. There's a happy medium.

Take care with being overly familiar with clients you don't know. Adding a hand on the shoulder, or a pat on the back is for those you know well. It's not for the client you've just signed on. Knowing when such additional non-verbal communication is appropriate is part of being able to read the bones of interpersonal niceties, especially in business.

Eye contact – handle with care

Making direct eye contact sends the message that you are genuinely interested in what the other person is saying. Of course, you should assess the length and intensity of the gaze. Sustained eye contact can be read as intimidation, or even sexual interest, so it's important that you look away occasionally, punctuating the action with a nod of the head, or other accompanying mannerisms to ensure it's not misunderstood as diminished interested.

How to Get Anybody to Do What You Want

How to Win Trust of a Person

This is one of the easiest tactics here, but it will make people respect you more and make them more partial to your influence. The simple fact is that a lot of people aren't used to honesty when they least expect it. More than that, the way to influence people — to really and honestly influence people — is to throw them off. If you want to influence people, you have to bewilder them and overpower them in terms of willpower. Consider it like a boxing match, you wait for your opponent to give you an opening before you throw a punch. However, here, you can create your own openings. You can give yourself an opening by doing things that people don't ordinarily expect, and this can earn their respect.

Being honest when people don't expect it is a huge part of successfully implementing this technique. Of course, you need to have a good sense of timing. Don't tell people that something is horrible or that their outfit looks bad or anything else explicitly rude. Rather, if you feel like everybody else is coddling them about something, be the opposition to the coddling. People know when they're being fed manure, even if it's just manure to make them feel better. Being somebody who sees through the manure will make them feel like you really understand them.

It's hard to define exactly what overt honesty means. It's a bit of a tricky definition in and of itself, after all. If you really want a definition of overt honesty, consider a situation where somebody is confiding something in you. They're nervous about some big life decision that's coming up. Overt honesty is not directing them to take one path or another, even if that's your ultimate goal in the conversation. Overt honesty is like them saying, "I just hope it will be okay," and then saying something like "It might not. You know that, and I'm sorry you're in this situation. It's awful. But..." and then proceed to carry on the conversation, slowly trying to swing them to your side through the use of other tactics.

The key here is letting them recognize that you understand them. Most people on the other end of the conversation would tell them "It will absolutely be okay," but you don't do that. You affirm their underlying fear (that it might not be okay), validate that fear by expressing it back to them, and make them feel like they should allow you to help them make a decision, even if it's not in a direct manner. This makes them subconsciously take your advice to heart than they would the advice of others.

It almost feels redundant to say this at this point, but it's of the utmost importance that you try to catch people off-guard. Whatever they're expecting, try to do the exact opposite of it. Not all the time, of course, but you're trying to make yourself look good, different, and trustworthy. In essence, you're trying to do what you can to make yourself look like you are somebody who can influence them.

One way to catch people off-guard is to maintain complete eye contact when you're telling them about something you genuinely care about or want to make it seem like you genuinely care about it. Use your intuition here, of course. Don't come off as creepy in the name of being influential. However, the right eye contact adds a degree of intensity and dominance to the conversation that's unparalleled, and if you practice it enough, you can easily make people come around to whatever you want them to do in tandem with the other things on this list.

Some of the ways that we've been using neuro-linguistic programming so far are setting up unique paradigms of honesty and outwardly charming personality traits. The combination of your general charm and your unique manner of speaking to people will make them see you as a trustworthy person.

Another way that we've discussed it is in the notion of taking yourself out of the equation and then framing the argument towards the thing that you want under the pretense of being objective. When you do this, you set things up such that the person starts to see you as impartial and objective. This is important because it programs people to value your opinion above the opinions of others because they see it as a more 'sound' idea than what others can offer.

So in the end, how can you take advantage of the concepts of neuro-linguistic programming to build your influence among people? There are a couple of different methods.

The first and foremost is to use it to establish an emotional connection between groups of people and yourself, or just one person and yourself. You need to start using terms like 'we' rather than 'I' to set up a subtle deference to either you or the group and a quiet sense of responsibility towards either you or the group. Don't completely replace 'I,' but do start referring to you and the person or people in question as a unit. This is an important part.

The second is to make yourself seem enigmatic. You do this by throwing people off-guard and coming off as someone who is very unique, as I've said before. Your goal isn't to ostracize or weird people out, though, so don't take it too far. What you ultimately want is for people to describe you positively, and that they see your personality and way of handling things as fundamentally distinct.

There are some other ways to use language to subtly turn people against things or in favor of things. These work best either from a false-objective standpoint (like the detached standpoint that we talked about before) or from a position where they see you as an influential person. There's actually a deep connotation with positive and negative words, such that even using positive or negative words in relation to something when somebody cares about your opinion can create a situation where they innately start to connect those positive or negative words to those concepts. For example, if you were trying to present one college as good and one college as bad, you could use vaguely good terms and phrasing to define the first while using vaguely bad terms and phrasing to define the second.

If you're too overt in this approach, people will realize that you're trying to make a contrast or a comparison between the two subjects. Rather, you need to use subtle phrasing. The first college, for example, may be 'affordable,' 'have great programs,' or 'a solid foundation.' The second college may be 'out of the way' or 'a little plain,' or you may just be 'a little worried about how good a degree from this one will look.'

It's with the use of these subtle phrases that you can begin to slowly program somebody's opinions regarding certain topics. Enough of this over time, and you can start to dramatically shift somebody's opinion on something.

Another way that you can program someone's opinions is to actually overstep the thing you don't like. For example, if you were trying to make an argument against something, you could say something so erroneously good about the opposition that the person will start to see it as ironic in their own mind and slowly see through what you presented. This is a very subtle and difficult thing to pull off, but it can be very rewarding when you do it right.

Remember, words have great power. One of the most important things that you can do is learn how to use this power to bend things in your favor.

Fear-Then-Relief Procedure

Plenty of marketers, brand managers, advertisers and business owners prey on the fears of consumers to manipulate them into buying from them. Make the person imagine the worst situation, followed by helping them feel relieved. This sneaky little trick will help you to get them to do precisely what you want them to.

For instance, you could say something like, "When I wore your dress for the prom night, I thought I heard a horrible sound of the dress tearing. I was sure I had torn your beautiful dress. However, I realized that it was just a video one of the girls was watching on her phone. Isn't that truly funny?" Oh and this reminds me, can I borrow the dress again for an upcoming weekend bash if you do not mind?

See what we did there? We simply took the person on a whirlwind of emotions from fear to immediate relief that the dress is still in good condition after all. They will be in a more positive and receptive frame of mind, which will increase your chances of having your way with them.

Why is fear such an effective tool in manipulation? Why do companies like to threaten you into compliance by asking you to buy something before stocks run out when they know full well that they have an entire warehouse of products? Why do manipulators like to instill fear in their victims? Fear is a negative emotion whose presence in the body inhibits rational decision making. Here's why:

When you are scared, there are only two thoughts on your mind: fight or flight. Nothing else. You really do not have the mind to start engaging in critical thinking or anything of the sort. Being scared or anxious sends your body into survival mode, and when you are in survival mode, you will choose one of two options that make the most sense to you. The neuroscience behind this is critical to understanding what makes fear such a favorite tool for manipulators. When your entire bodily systems are in that flight-or-flight response mode, your critical thinking circuitry is bypassed. In short, your brain does not have the intention to start processing the tiny details at the moment. So, instead of utilizing the more analytical neocortex to think, you rely on the primitive limbic system. Later on, when you are in a more relaxed state, your critical thinking capability is activated, and you start to wonder why you made that particular decision when in fact there were other options to explore.

At all times, be careful of anyone who cries wolf. They might be trying to distract you from the other options that are available to be explored in your decision-making. At the same time, you must take advantage of the opportunity presented by fear to influence other people. There are various ways of taking advantage of fear in situations. For a start, you can exaggerate a situation and make it seem far worse than it is. Let's say you are a manager and you catch this one employee skipping work without official leave. It's a slow day anyway, and there's not much work to be done--but they know they should not be skipping work, and you intend to take full advantage of this situation.

What to do? For a start, you need to make this seem like the biggest deal of the century. How dare they hide from work and expect to receive a paycheck at the end of the month? Do they know what would happen if this got to the other bosses? You might even want to mention that they have put you in a really awkward position by engaging in such a foolish act. Now that you have got your employee shaking in their boots (assuming that they really need the job and the paycheck) ask them whether they would be willing to work the weekend shift to make up for this lost time, in exchange for a slap on the wrist. The employee will most likely say yes. They have not had time to even come up with a good lie because their minds are in flight or fight mode. You'll then go on about your day happily knowing full well that you do not have to work the weekend shift and can instead spend the day doing what you truly enjoy.

Aside from exaggerating the truth, you can instill fear by spreading blatant lies. This approach has worked since time immemorial and continues to be effective to date. Using the same example of a manager, let's assume you have noticed that the employees are slacking in their duties, including coming in late for work and generally being lazy. You have tried all means to motivate them, and nothing seems to be working. What can you do? Consider this: find the one employee with the loosest mouth and let it slip that there will be an impromptu performance review by management sometime soon. This loose-lipped employee will do the legwork for you and ensure that the entire rumor mill knows what's about to happen. You will begin to notice that your employees are working harder and coming to work earlier because they are fearful of the consequences of facing management.

Fear in manipulation works best where the party that is being manipulated stands to lose or miss out on something. You must determine that whatever carrot you are dangling in front of your victim is worth their attention. Otherwise there will be no interest and consequently, no success in your manipulation efforts. If you know what makes someone tick, you will always know what buttons to push to make them fearful.

Making You Feel Guilty: Social Exchange

You have heard of mind games. You have surely played them before and had them played on you. You can use mind games as an effective persuasion tool when you know what to do and when. There are numerous techniques that are effective, and they are not that difficult to learn. This means that once you know what they are, you can start utilizing mind games right away to start getting what you want.

Kick Me

This likely reminds you of that game when you were a kid where you put a sign on someone's back that read "kick me." This is similar. You want to make yourself look like someone that deserves pity. Once you get pity from someone, it is easier to get them to do what you want. You can use this for just about anything in life from getting someone to allow you to apologize to getting a boss to give you a promotion once you get really good at it.

Now That I've Got You

This is a game that you will use when you want to show a person you are winning and better. You can also use it when you are angry and want to justify it. For example, your friend had a party, but he neglected to invite you. So, you decide to host a party the following weekend with the intent to just not invite him. This game basically has you working to one up another person to get them to give in and give you what you want.

You Made Me Do It

This is another one you used during childhood and you likely did not even realize at the time that it was a type of mind game. This is a game that works to make another person feel guilty while simultaneously absolving you of any responsibility for your actions. For example, you want to be left alone. However, someone comes in the room to ask you a question. As a result, you are startled and drop your beverage. You tell that person that they made you drop your beverage.

If It Weren't for You

This is another mind game that is used to absolve yourself of any guilt for something you might have done. With this type of game, you essentially create a scenario that allows you to put guilt onto someone. This gives you an array of advantages. When a person is feeling guilty about something, they are more vulnerable to suggestion. For example, you are unable to go to work for whatever reason. You find a way to blame your spouse for this and make them feel guilty. As a result, you are able to coerce your spouse into making you a meal or buying you something.

Let You Both Fight

The purpose of this mind game is to share blame, control other people and even make yourself seem like a good friend. In most cases, this is a mind game that women will play, but it is becoming more common among men. For example, a person knows that two people are attracted to them. This person then talks both of the interested parties into fighting with one another to basically win their heart. This is basically a type of transaction, however, at the end of the game, both interested parties are usually left without anyone.

RAPO

This mind game can be a major ego boost, give a sense of satisfaction and increase how desirable you see yourself to be. It is a type of social game in which you essentially convince a person to pursue you. You convince them in a way that is not obvious to them, so they do not even know what it is happening. How you choose to convince them is flexible and really dependent on your preferences and what it takes to get into the subconscious of the person you are seeking to lure. What is good about this game is that it generally does not take long to put into practice.

Perversion

The purpose of this game is to avoid responsibility and garner sympathy. Basically, this mind game is used to seduce another person. You cause them to feel guilty if they are not fulfilling your romantic needs. You talk about a bad past relationship, whether it was real or not, to first get sympathy from them. Then, once they essentially soften to the idea of fulfilling your desires, you go in and take what you want. If they are still resistant, you cause them to feel guilty to ultimately get what you want.

Clever Me

This one improves your identity, social capital, attention and ego. You do something to show someone what you are great at and you want the entire world to know that you are awesome at this specific thing. You manipulate the situation to make sure that someone will learn about your skill. You get attention from them and they tell others. Before you know it, your skill or talent is being spread around and a lot of people are coming to you to pay you a compliment.

Wooden Leg

This is a game people play for sympathy, as a plea of insanity or to avoid responsibility. You have likely heard the saying that you can only expect so much from a person who has a wooden leg. This game is built upon this saying. Basically, you use a perceived shortfall or disability to gain sympathy and make your actions seem justified. For example, you just cheated on your spouse and he or she found out. You would say something like, "well, my parents had a bad marriage, so what do you expect of me?". They then start to give you sympathy and you are absolved of your guilt.

The Double Request

This is a common mind game among those who want something big but know that they will not get it just asking for it. For example, you ask for a new expensive watch, but you really want a new jacket that tends to be less expensive. You mention both items, but you make it seem like the watch is what you truly desire. In the end, the friend you are talking to remembers that the jacket was cheaper and also something that you wanted, so they buy it. You end up getting the jacket you wanted from the start.

You're a Good Person

This is a common mind game to play when you want to get something out of someone that they are not normally asked. When you start the conversation by telling them that they are a good person, they are getting recognition and an ego boost from you. This already softens them and makes them more prone to give you exactly what you want. Once you see that their body language is softer or even just neutral, you want to go in and ask for what you want.

Conclusion

You will agree with the assessment that manipulation is everywhere in our daily lives. Even while you sleep, there is a brand somewhere that is looking to unleash their manipulative marketing campaign with the goal of making you spend your money. While you slave away at work at the mercy of your boss, there is often no guarantee that you will get a promotion. In your personal relationships, there is probably someone who is pretending to be your friend but is only looking out for themselves. It almost seems like whichever way you turn, there is someone waiting to influence your next move. This can be quite overwhelming.

Being manipulated does not feel good. Knowing that everything you thought was true was an altered reality created by a manipulative person makes you feel betrayed and, often times, stupid. You wonder why you did not see the red flags and what you could have done differently. The truth of the matter is that however smart you think you are, there is always someone who believes they can outsmart you. Enter your new manipulation methods.

You do not have to sit back and watch other people take control and get what you want when you can do it yourself. Influencing other people into fulfilling your desires is well within your reach if you internalize and incorporate the teachings and methods of this book. It might seem like an uphill climb, especially if you are used to giving other people what they want and getting nothing in return, but it really is not. Learning how to manipulate people is not something that should overwhelm you. It only feels overwhelming now because you are learning all these new things all at once. With time and practice, the things you have learned will become second nature. You will find yourself smiling and flirting without even thinking about it.

Start the work from within--working on your body language, presentation, communication techniques--and then apply the outcome to the external environment. You will be surprised how much more you can gain from people and the world around you if you subtly manipulate them. Becoming a master manipulator will take you longer than a few days, but it will be worth the work and the wait. Remember, as long as you are not hurting anyone who does not deserve to be hurt, you are well within your rights to manipulate your way to the success that you have always envisioned for yourself!

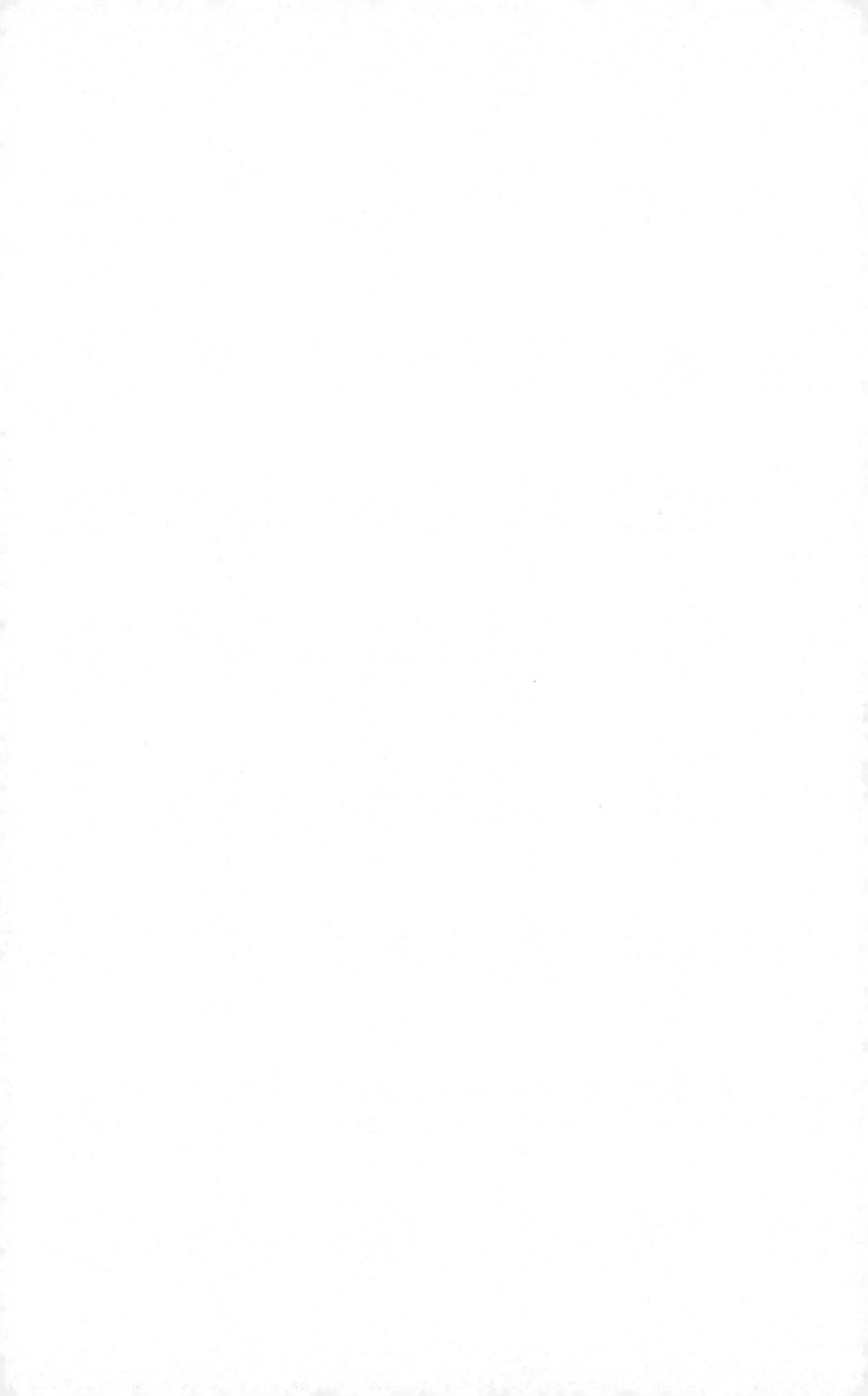

Made in the USA
Columbia, SC
29 April 2020